"Dr. Samadi has a passion for helping and in particular a passion for helping men. We are not easy. I too am a physician, but I am also a patient with prostate cancer. So I understand men's health from the perspective of caretaker and patient. Dr. Samadi has created a very digestible source from which we can easily access some of the most important priorities for men's health and the treatment of common men's medical conditions. An excellent resource that is not to be missed by a true leader in men's health."

—Dr. Drew Pinsky
Internist and addictionologist

"Dr. Samadi is a physician and specialist with impeccable credentials who writes in a clear, understandable style and offers practical recommendations for men to improve their health. Men fall behind women in terms of both health and life expectancy. Dr. Samadi strikes a blow for equality by leveling the playing field."

—Dinesh D'Souza
Author and filmmaker

"As a woman and a health expert, I am impressed with the message this book offers men. It will enable them to take charge of their health, reduce the risks of cancer and other urological problems, manage sexual performance issues, and live longer, happier lives. Dr. Samadi's personal story is riveting, and his expertise, gained at world-class institutions such as Memorial Sloan Kettering in New York City and Henri Mondor Hospital in Paris, is impressive."

—Betsy McCaughey, PhD, former lieutenant governor of New York State
Chairman, Committee to Reduce Infection Deaths

"Few know medicine like Dr. Samadi, the 'ultimate' expert when it comes to men's health. This book is a must-read for every man and the women who love them."

—Christopher Ruddy
CEO, Newsmax Media

"The hallmark of men's health is that the life expectancy of men is shorter than women. Addressing the unmet need to improve men's health, Dr. Samadi's book, *The Ultimate MANual*, combines science with simplicity, evidence with practicality, and details with common sense. It is a must-read for men of all ages. This fantastic book presents a comprehensive approach, not only explaining what to do when sick but how to improve and maintain health when healthy."

—Ridwan Shabsigh, MD, FACS
Past president, International Society of Men's Health
Editor-in-chief, *Journal of Men's Health*

THE ULTIMATE
MANUAL

Dr. Samadi's Guide to
Men's Health and Wellness

David Samadi, MD

www.prostatecancer911.com
www.roboticoncology.com

Cover design: Alan Barnett, www.alanbarnett.com
Cover photo: Courtesy of MD News
Book design: Alan Barnett, www.alanbarnett.com
Illustrations: Gail Bean, www.gailbeanfineart.com
Editor: Christina Roth, www.christinarotheditorial.com

Library of Congress Control Number: 2020916161

ISBN 978-1-7352969-0-6

Printed in the United States of America

To the thousands of men I've treated and their families,
continually inspiring me to work towards quality
healthcare for all men everywhere

CONTENTS

FOREWORD

I first met Dr. Samadi in person in 2012. He had had a long and illustrious career at some of the top New York City hospitals and was renowned for his superlative robotic radical prostatectomy technique and results. Patients from Australia to Zimbabwe were seeking his expertise. Most were identifying him not from any appreciable social media presence or advertising but from old-fashioned word-of-mouth recommendation by the multitudes of satisfied American and international patients. In addition, his peer-reviewed publications were bolstering his reputation with his colleagues, resulting in his umpteen invitations to international urologic conventions, where he taught his craft of perfecting robotic radical prostatectomy with the best functional results ever published, particularly in preserving both sexual function and urinary continence. It was then that I made it my quest to create the opportunity for us to work together.

I knew where he lived and was going to make every effort to get him to move his practice to our hospital, including enticing him with proximity to home. It did not hurt that our hospital, St. Francis Hospital in Roslyn, New York, is a gem and well known in the New York Metro area as one of the safest and best overall hospitals to receive and deliver care. Over the next six years, I followed his career and frequently saw his appearances on national television, where he opined on men's health matters in his typically eloquent, insightful, and kind manner.

Fast-forward to 2019, and we made it happen—and I could not be happier. David is now our Director of Men's Health and Urologic Oncology. Being in direct, daily contact with him has reaffirmed my esteem for a person at the helm of his craft. David embodies the tenets of the famous physician Maimonides, who espoused the science of medicine in the context of human kindness, humility, and individual attention to detail. He is supremely driven to do what is right for his patients and has a sincere desire to spread his knowledge and care to a wider audience than most of us lesser physicians can achieve.

The authorship of this wonderful "MANual" is the embodiment of his commitment to help that wider audience. In reading this treatise, I am amazed by his organization of thought, ease of explaining sometimes complex concepts, and outstanding advice that, if we took, would lead to a more vibrant, healthful, and longer life.

I am proud to call David Samadi, MD my friend and even prouder to have him as a colleague and clinical resource in men's health. His contributions as a resource to our community's health and wellness are immeasurable.

Gary R. Gecelter, MD, FACS, FACG
Chairman, Department of Surgery
St. Francis Hospital, Roslyn, New York
August 2020

PREFACE

As a urologist, I have a unique opportunity to not only care for issues related to a man's urinary tract and reproductive system but also to coordinate care to address many other health problems I come across daily. We'll discuss this concept later. For now, I want to share the story of my personal journey to becoming a urologist, a subspecialty that you will become much more familiar with in this book.

It begins with where I was born—Iran. Iran is one of the world's oldest civilizations. Known throughout most of history as Persia, its borders changed regularly during its early years, first because the nomadic tribes who lived there were constantly on the move, and later because the country was routinely overrun, invaded, and occupied by Arabs, Turks, Mongols, Brits, Russians, and others—all anxious to get their hands on this vast, largely undeveloped country that enjoyed a strategic location in the Middle East.

I was born and raised as a Jew living in the Persian Jewish community in Tehran, Iran. As a child, I attended a Western-style school run by the Don Bosco Catholic order, captained the soccer team, attended temple on the High Holy Days, and enjoyed Friday night Shabbat dinners with my parents, siblings, and extended family of aunts, uncles, and cousins. Life was very good, and I saw myself living the rest of my days in Iran.

However, life has a way of abruptly changing well-thought-out plans. My vision for my future would take a dramatic turn due to turmoil in my native country. The Islamic Revolution in 1979 changed everything in the world I knew and was a defining, unexpected moment in time that would eventually lead me to the United States. At the age of fifteen, I was forced to flee the country I loved with my younger brother, Dan, leaving behind our parents and younger sister, Hedieh. For the next eight years, my brother and I lived among strangers in Belgium, London, and finally the United States, whose shores we arrived on in 1984. This period of time was a testing ground of sorts, forcing both my brother and me to grow up fast as we struggled with the loneliness of being separated from our beloved family. Finally, in 1990, my parents and younger sister were able to move to the US, where all of us have become citizens and deeply appreciate and love this country we now call home. Dan is a now a successful ear, nose, and throat (ENT) doctor, and Hedieh has a busy career as a dentist. My parents are alive and well, living happily on Long Island where they enjoy seeing their children and grandchildren frequently.

They say adversity defines your character and values in life. Even though I went through intense hardship and difficulties, I am eternally grateful for how it lit the fire of motivation and desire to succeed by giving back to others in need in any way I could. I knew that my parents sacrificed a great deal for me and Dan, and we both wanted to honor them by making them proud of us. My dear mother was especially instrumental with her emphasis on education, which would eventually play a pivotal role in opening doors to our future careers. There is no way I can ever repay her or my beloved father for their enduring love and guidance during my childhood. Thanks to my values-focused upbringing, my personal experiences and everything I've learned plays directly into how I perform my job as a doctor and surgeon in the operating room. My patients' safety, outcomes, and results are always a top priority—I will always protect my patients and their families. I consider myself highly involved in the emotional well-being of each patient I see and that of their partner and family. The doctor-patient relationship has to be based on trust and understanding. When my patients feel I am being genuine in providing the very best possible medical treatment they require, this is a huge step in gaining their confidence in my abilities to get them well. That alone is such a necessary part of providing healthcare. When my patients come to me for their medical needs, they become a part of my family, and I want them to know that.

When Dan and I arrived in Roslyn, New York, back in 1984, we found ourselves much happier. Even though our love of Iran was still strong and the loneliness for our family only grew, the ability to live in this beautiful, free country is a gift I will always cherish. I can proudly say I am living the American dream. In those early years of living in this great nation, Dan and I found ourselves excelling in high school with dreams of becoming doctors. We were both accepted into medical schools: my acceptance was with Stony Brook School of Medicine, and Dan's was with New York University.

After graduating from Stony Brook, I began my formal training in urology, starting in 1994 with a six-year surgical residency at New York City's Montefiore Medical Center and its two affiliated hospitals, Albert Einstein College of

Medicine and Jacobi Medical Center. The Montefiore program included a six-month rotation in urology surgery at Memorial Sloan Kettering Cancer Center which included an oncology fellowship in urology. It was while I was at Sloan Kettering that I received a second fellowship in robotic radical prostatectomy to study at Henri Mondor Hospital in Paris. My mentor and a pioneer in the field at that time was Dr. Claude Abbou, who introduced me to laparoscopic surgery. This was where I got my first glimpse of the course of my future, when in 2001 a da Vinci robotic surgical system was sent to Paris. Dr. Abbou had me assist him in one of the first eleven robotic laparoscopic prostatectomies in the world.

In 2002, I returned to New York, where I joined the staff at Columbia-Presbyterian Hospital. I spent five years there heading up the laparoscopic surgery unit in the department of urology. It was during this time I introduced the department to a state-of-the-art da Vinci robotic surgical system. In May 2007, my team moved to Mount Sinai Medical Center, where I was named the chief of robotics and minimally invasive surgery. By 2013, I had become the chairman of urology and the chief of robotic surgery at Lenox Hill Hospital and was named to the prestigious Castle Connolly America's Top Doctors and *New York Magazine*'s Best Doctors List. Currently, I am Director of Men's Health and Urologic Oncology at St. Francis Hospital, Roslyn, New York.

Over the course of my medical career, I have had the good fortune of being able to share and educate others on my knowledge of men's health and urology. I've written many publications and have spoken many times across the nation and abroad.

My most unusual and rather unexpected bit of good luck is what has taken me from doing surgery to also becoming a contributor and medical consultant for broadcast news. From repeated appearances on *Fox & Friends* and Newsmax to a regular stint on *Sunday Housecall,* I've been able to share my knowledge and expertise on a variety of health topics. I even did a guest cameo on *Law & Order.* My acting abilities may be limited, but luckily the role I played was a urologist raising awareness of prostate cancer.

Some people have asked why I decided to go into urology. For as long as I can remember, I knew I wanted to help people, and what better way than to become a doctor? The road to getting an MD behind your name takes years of diligent study and determination, and I had plenty of both. The long hours, difficult decisions that must be made daily, and hard work are well worth the tremendous effort when you witness people regaining good health and improved quality of life.

My true passion for urology stems from a relentless ambition to improve men's health, especially when it comes to fighting prostate cancer. When I was in medical school, I was scheduled one day to observe a cardiac surgery. However, it was cancelled at the last moment. Instead, I watched a prostate cancer surgery for the first time. Standing next to the surgeon and watching him navigate around such a small area of the body was fascinating. I instantly knew prostate and men's health was my calling in medicine. I've never regretted my decision.

Today, I have enjoyed a long career of helping thousands of men and their families with various urological issues. My urology specialty is in urologic oncology, which emphasizes diagnosing and treating prostate cancer. To be able to establish lifelong ties with these men and their partners is a true privilege. These men are more than just patients—they are part of my extended family.

My goal in writing this book is to help even more men like you improve their health and, in turn, their quality of life. I'm excited to be a guide along your journey toward better health—for you, for those you love, and for others who may be inspired by your journey.

Dr. David Samadi
New York City

ACKNOWLEDGMENTS

Writing a book is comparable to practicing medicine. Rarely is it practiced without others being involved, each having their own special role. It takes a team effort to make it happen and get the best result. I've learned that when composing a book, you draw upon your experiences of interacting with those who've been either mentors, healthcare professionals, patients, dear friends, or beloved family members.

I want to start by extending my most heartfelt thanks to my immediate family, who've made the greatest sacrifice of tolerating my long work hours while supporting and encouraging me to follow my dreams. I especially thank my beautiful and understanding wife, Sahar, whose unconditional love and support kept me, our children, and our home in order. I also want to thank my two wonderful children, Jasmine and Alex, whom I love more than they will ever know. They are my life's greatest blessings.

My parents, I cannot thank you enough for the opportunities you've provided me and the difference you've made in my life. Your love, your support, and the sacrifices you made for me and my brother and sister will never be forgotten. I also need to extend my love and gratitude to my brother, Daniel, and my sister, Hedieh—our bond will never be broken.

Next, I extend my deepest gratitude and praise for all the mentors I've been fortunate enough to have guided me along my journey as a physician. From teachers to fellow doctors to colleagues, your tireless work, loads of energy, and unfailing encouragement is what kept me pursuing my goal of helping others reach good health and my dream of becoming a doctor.

Finally I want to recognize my top-notch surgical team and office staff by extending my sincere thanks for standing by me all these years to help care for our patients. I could not have done it without any of you.

INTRODUCTION

Let's begin with good news first—men are living much longer than in years past. Back in 1900, most babies were lucky if they made it to the age of fifty. Thanks to vast improvements in modern medical technology, life-extending medications, earlier and enhanced screenings for diseases, and public health campaigns, all of us have enjoyed and benefited from a longer life span.

Are you ready for the not-so-good news? While men may be living longer, are they necessarily living healthier? That's a question I have asked myself many times over the course of my medical career. We all know a stubborn man who refuses to go to the doctor, right? This may be one reason why men have a shorter life expectancy than women. In 2018, the latest information from the National Center for Health Statistics, total life expectancy at birth was 78.7 years in the United States. Women fared better, with a life expectancy of 81.2 years, while men's life expectancy barely increased from 76.1 years in 2016 to 76.2 in 2018.[1] In other words, a woman living in the US can expect to live a full five years longer than a man living in the same country.

This lower life expectancy in men is also seen throughout the rest of the world. In the 2016 World Health Statistics, men had a shorter life expectancy than women in all countries. On average, men's life expectancy at birth was six years shorter than that of women.[2]

Society as a whole likes to think of men as strong, virile, in control, and full of stamina and endurance. There are many men who can be described this way. But plenty of other men do not fit that description. Regardless of the cause of death, men have a higher mortality rate than women. Chronic disease such as heart disease, hypertension, diabetes, and cancer all affect men at both higher morbidity and mortality rates than women. Besides diseases, men may be more likely to indulge in lifestyle choices leading to poor health, including smoking, excessive alcohol consumption, illegal drug use, a sedentary lifestyle, obesity, poor eating habits, and other high-risk behaviors.

What is missing for men when it comes to the disparity between their health and women's health? Is it possible men fail to see a doctor when they are physically or mentally suffering, resulting in a worse outcome? And if so, why?

Comparing how men and women approach healthcare is like comparing apples to oranges. Women generally take a more pragmatic approach, asking numerous and detailed questions. I see this all the time in my practice. If a man is by himself, the visit is much shorter than if his wife or girlfriend comes along, usually with a long list of questions, which I welcome. For instance, my specialty is taking care of men with prostate cancer—the ultimate equal opportunity disease that impacts not only the men who get it but the women who share lives with them. The men who come to see me bring their prostates, but their wives or girlfriends bring notebooks filled with questions.

Women approach healthcare the right way—take good care of yourself before health issues happen. Even studies have found women are more likely to seek out healthcare than men are.[3] Men can learn a thing or two from women in this respect.

Maybe women take this proactive approach because they have built relationships with their physicians—they see them frequently during their reproductive years and are accustomed to screenings like Pap smears starting early in life. Men tend to feel uncomfortable about screenings, often resisting routine invasive exams such as digital rectal exams. Men may also fear receiving news of a serious diagnosis. In a 2016 online survey, more than 20 percent of men said finding out they might have a health problem was a roadblock to scheduling an annual exam.[4] But I'm here to tell men that waiting until symptoms get worse is not a good health plan.

As a urologist and a man who predominantly sees male patients, I uniquely understand men. Over my seventeen-year career, I've had the opportunity to listen and talk with thousands of my male patients and their significant others. I've seen and attended to plenty of men who have neglected their health over the years.

The optimal time for practicing good health habits is early in life.

For some reason, men often ignore that message. Poor food choices, lack of exercise, tobacco use, one too many late nights, or one too many alcoholic beverages puts a man's health at risk. Men simply tend to put their health last on their to-do list—as long as they can keep working and being productive, they often don't consider the health risks their neglect causes.

When men live by the "don't fix it until it's broke" mantra, they create a predicament. They may find themselves in their forties, fifties, and beyond receiving a diagnosis of a "silent" disease such as coronary heart disease, prostate cancer, or kidney disease, each potentially lowering their life span by years. Or they may become frustrated or worried over bedroom activities and end up getting diagnosed with erectile dysfunction or low testosterone. Mr. Happy not working like he used to is often what motivates men to come see me in the first place.

While many doctors state they are in healthcare, the truth is most of us are in *disease* care, especially regarding men. In other words, the vast majority of our male patients come to us because they are sick or have medical conditions affecting their health; rarely is their initial visit a discussion totally focused on getting and staying healthy. Too bad that's not the case.

My educational background includes an oncology fellowship in urology at Memorial Sloan Kettering Cancer Center and a robotic prostatectomy fellowship at Henri Mondor Hospital in France. As a urologic oncologist expert and robotic surgeon, over the years I've witnessed men who waited too long to see a doctor before their prostate cancer spread, making it more difficult to manage. If they had taken steps to take charge of their health throughout their life, they likely would have had a different outcome.

That's why I am writing this book. The men I see every day want and deserve excellent healthcare. Urology is my specialty, yet many medical issues involve other areas of the male body that affect how their urinary system functions. Male-specific issues such as erectile dysfunction, premature ejaculation, testosterone deficiency, and prostate and testicular cancer are associated with cardiovascular risk factors and can be predictors of other medical conditions, such as diabetes, hypertension, hyperlipidemia (high cholesterol), and angina. While these male-specific issues may not contribute significantly to a man's mortality, they do and can adversely affect a man's quality of life.

This is where doctors can learn a thing or two from women—we need to think differently on how we take care of men. When we are proactive, the men we care for will always get a better return on the investment in their health. Shouldn't that always be our goal?

My goal for every patient I see is to assess their overall health, from head to toe. While I am a board-certified urologist and a specialist in diagnosing and treating urologic conditions, I want men to pay attention to their total body by understanding how to get and stay healthy. Men who take good care of themselves feel better, look better, and greatly improve their sexual health. When bedroom activities are going great, there's no need to rock the boat by dismissing your health.

By reading this book, you and your partner will discover how achieving your best health is within your reach. You are the expert of your body, and you hold the key to unlocking its full potential by making healthy lifestyle changes. I will guide you on your journey toward becoming the healthy man you are meant to be. Aside from helping men catch up with women on adding years to their life, I'll also show you how to add more life to your years—which is even more important. More energy, better sleep, less stress, and an active and fulfilled sex life—what else could a man ask for?

This book is divided into four parts, so here's what you can expect:

Part 1 will pull back the curtain on the state of men's health. How do men and women approach healthcare differently and why? What are the top health risks and diseases affecting men?

Part 2 will take an in-depth look at the specific urinary issues men face—prostate, penis, testicular, bladder, and kidney issues; other conditions affecting the penis; and factors negatively affecting a man's sexual functioning, including ways to overcome them for a satisfying love life.

Part 3 will tackle the necessary lifestyle habits all men should adopt—eating a healthy diet, exercising regularly, reducing stress, getting a better night's sleep, and refraining from illicit substances. This section will also review not only Western medicine but also Eastern medicines like herbs and supplements.

Part 4 is a compilation of recipes containing nutrients especially beneficial for men, complete with nutritional information. Whether you're a gourmet cook or a newbie to preparing meals, you will find simple, delicious, and nutritious options for every meal and for snacks. This section will also include a two-week meal plan to help you get started on better eating habits.

Like the saying goes, health is wealth. You are in charge of your health, and you get to decide how to take care of yourself. Your decisions throughout life all add up to whether you are wealthy in your overall health and well-being.

Ready to lead a prosperous life filled with fantastic physical, emotional, and mental health? Then let's get started on your journey to becoming an *ultimate man*.

PART 1

The State of Men's Health

CHAPTER 1

Saving Lives, One Man at a Time

Men, I'm here for you. As a urologist, I love my job treating and taking care of men. I'm dedicated to saving men's lives, literally. My top priority is for every man to experience his best health at all stages of his life. When men adopt and practice good health habits, starting as early as their teens, they're making an investment in their long-term health with a significant payout of quality-of-life dividends.

But it's the women in your life who can benefit from much of what I'll discuss in this chapter. These women include your wives, girlfriends, mother, sisters, daughters, and all women who love you and only want the best for you. Statistics show women make 80 percent of the medical decisions in a household.[1] That's why I need to recruit an army of women who encourage men to live healthier lives. Women are simply better advocates of their families' health. They are very good at prioritizing health. They get fired up on overseeing not only their own well-being but also the well-being of all men in their lives, from their fathers to their sons and husbands.

Before I get too deep into this chapter, let's take a look at the differences between men and women that provide a little context. Do you remember the book *Men Are from Mars, Women Are from Venus* by John Gray, PhD? This 1992 bestseller boldly and decisively struck a nerve when it addressed common conflicts between men and women and how we each react differently to them. Because of these differences between us, it may sometimes feel as if we come from two different planets.

Have you ever gone shopping for clothes with your wife or girlfriend? All you want is a pair of pants. You know which store you want to buy them from and where they are in the store. This trip should be easy, right? Wrong, not if you're shopping with a woman. The way women tend to shop is one example of how they make decisions differently than men do. What should be an easy in-and-out shopping trip might turn into a much longer and more expensive excursion than you were planning. The following illustration speaks a million words to my point:

Go to the Mall to Buy a Shirt

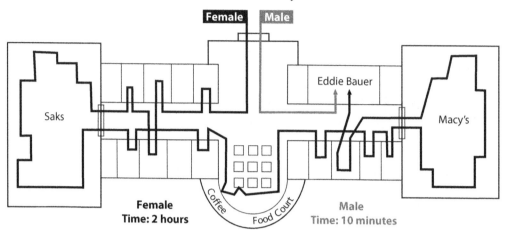

Now, I have the utmost respect for women. I strongly value their intelligence, insight, and sensitivity and believe we as men can learn a great deal from it. My point with the illustration is to demonstrate that women explore all options before making a decision. They compare and contrast what looks good and what doesn't, what to buy and what to put back on the rack. This same instinctual method is also how women tend to approach healthcare decisions, including who should be the family primary care physician and what pharmacy to use. It's probably also your wife who keeps accurate records of family members' immunizations and upcoming checkups or preventive screening tests. Thanks to women's detail-oriented brains and organizational skills that allow them to take charge of their family's medical needs, each family member benefits from significantly improved health and well-being and increased longevity.

What Women Should Know about Men's Health

Men's health or lack thereof is a real issue. Every day I see men who have neglected their health for a long time. I have cared for men in their forties, fifties, and older who have not visited a doctor since childhood. Many men are hard-pressed to even remember their primary care physician's name when filling out medical forms. In fact, if it weren't for my take-charge pragmatic wife, even I would be a bad patient.

Not only will neglect put men's health at risk, but when men are sick or inflicted with a disease, it affects the women in their lives as well. Caring for anyone who needs extra attention automatically adds stress, anxiety, and possible financial burdens to those women, and it gives them less time to pay attention to their own health. But together, we can turn that around. When men begin to make changes to improve their health with the women they love cheering them on, it makes a tremendous difference for both of you.

So, why do men have this natural tendency to put their health last? Why would a man avoid regular checkups or not do what it takes to be healthy?

One big reason men neglect their health is that life gets busy. There are bills to pay, food to put on the table, and not enough time to think about themselves. Therefore, going to the doctor is a waste of time, especially for regular screenings—who wants to sit in a waiting room thumbing through old magazines or watching HGTV?

I can attest from years of experience that a consultation with a man takes less time than a woman's visit with her doctor. Not because men are healthier or have fewer medical concerns, but primarily by their own choosing. Men are often in and out of the exam room within a matter of minutes. They provide few specifics and usually answer the doctor's questions with a simple yes or no. Men also ask few questions and want just the facts without going into detail. They often figure the less time spent perched on the exam table, the better.

Another big one is that men are problem-solvers. How many times has your wife or significant other felt frustrated when you're lost and won't ask for directions? Or when you refuse to see a doctor when you aren't feeling well? Most people would say these frustrations exist because women are emotional while men are logical. But logically speaking, if a man knows he's not feeling well, why wouldn't he seek a doctor's help to figure it out? Because he'd rather handle it himself than be bothered seeing a doctor who will try to educate or instruct him on a health issue.

Remember boys who couldn't sit still in school? They wanted to move around, experiment, and find solutions for themselves. Just because a man has grown up doesn't mean that restless boy inside is gone. Men like to figure out what the problem is on their own, so going to the doctor might humiliate them and make them feel like a loser.

And that brings us to another reason men avoid the doctor—they love being a winner. Many men thrive on success. That's why so many men enjoy sports and why they admire winning teams. Men having a health problem does not feel successful. If a man with this mindset is pressured to see a doctor, it can backfire with him avoiding the situation even further.

And of course, men don't like to be told what to do. They figure they've come this far in life without paying attention to their health or seeing a doctor. Besides, what if the doctor does find something wrong? It likely will make him feel vulnerable and that he needs to change. Change is difficult. Most men want to act strong, hoping time heals all things. But sticking your head in the sand and pretending like a health complication doesn't exist doesn't help anyone avoid it.

Likely, the most basic reason men are reluctant to go see the doctor is they will feel out of control. In case you haven't noticed, men like to be in control. From controlling the TV remote to deciding what restaurant to eat at, feeling in control makes men feel confident and self-assured.

Whatever the reason men avoid the doctor, a common attitude might include, "See a doctor? What do you think I am, sick?"

How many men do you know who suffered a serious injury but did not see a doctor for it? They dug in their heels, refusing to get the injury treated and adamantly believing they could deal with it on their own. Maybe they got lucky and it did heal. Or maybe the wound became infected, forcing them to seek medical help and leading to a longer, more complicated recovery. Why trust luck when you can't guarantee it will always be on your side, though?

Men should remember that no matter their age, none of us is invincible. For example, I had a patient in his early twenties who had originally gone to the doctor for episodes of blood in his urine. The doctor dismissed him, saying he was too young to have anything serious associated with this symptom. Six months later, this same young man was still experiencing bloody urine and made an appointment with me. After a thorough examination and diagnostic testing, the final conclusion was not what any of us expected—a large bladder cancer, very unusual for someone so young.

No one should ever take their youth or health for granted. While serious medical conditions can strike unexpectedly at any age, there's a greater chance of beating them back when caught early.

The Impact of the 2020 Coronavirus Pandemic on Men

I would be remiss not to mention the enormous impact of a novel coronavirus that started in Wuhan, China, in late 2019 that would greatly impact men's health. Caused by SARS-CoV-2, the World Health Organization (WHO) gave it the acronym COVID-19, which stands for **co**rona**vi**rus **d**isease 20**19**. As this book was being written, the unprecedented, historic pandemic was sweeping around the globe, shutting down businesses and leaving them in financial ruin while claiming far too many lives. COVID-19 posed a great danger for everyone, especially the elderly. However, it also took a noticeable and concerning toll on men. Not only did men of all ages contract the illness at a higher rate than women, but they were also more likely to have severe illness or die from it.

This was not the first time men were hit hard by a pandemic infectious disease. In 2003, even though more women than men were infected by the SARS outbreak, the death rate among men was significantly higher than women's. The MERS outbreak in the Middle East in 2012 infected men at a rate of 32 percent compared to 28.5 percent of women.[2]

Why would men be more vulnerable to developing more severe cases of and dying from an infectious disease? Perhaps as more data is gathered after COVID-19 has moved on, there will be a clearer answer. Until then, here are interesting possibilities of why this virus profoundly attacked men more than women:

- It's speculative, but despite men's tough exterior, our immune response against viral infections may be weaker than women's. Women appear to have a stronger immune response, reducing their susceptibility to viral infections. Thanks to their genetic makeup—women have two X chromosomes, men have one X and one Y chromosome—women may have a wider diversity of immune response.

- Men, especially those sixty-five and older or living in a long-term care facility, had far worse outcomes. If these same men had preexisting uncontrolled health conditions, including heart disease, diabetes, obesity, chronic lung disease, asthma, liver disease, chronic kidney disease, or being immunocompromised, they also paid a dire price. This same pattern was also similar to that of the MERS outbreak. Men during that illness who had chronic comorbidities (two or more chronic medical conditions simultaneously) tended to have weaker immune functioning and died at higher rates.[3]

- While smoking rates have gone down, US men still outpace women in lighting up (15.6 percent versus 12.0 percent).[4] Smokers have higher rates of pneumonia and chronic obstructive pulmonary disease (COPD), which increases the severity and complications of an infectious disease.

- Remember, there are plenty of men who simply don't like going to a doctor.[5] They will delay treatment, ignore symptoms, or be in denial when feeling sick. Men who wait too long before they are properly diagnosed and treated generally face a worse outcome.

- During the coronavirus pandemic, some men displayed a false sense of security, believing they could "tough it out" or that it wasn't as bad as believed. These men may have also ignored safety recommendations such as frequent handwashing or maintaining social distancing to protect themselves and others from contracting the virus.

- Black men disproportionately were disadvantaged by both contracting and dying from COVID-19 at higher rates.[6] Theories at this time blame several factors: poverty, segregation, crowded living conditions, or limited access to, putting off, or avoiding seeking healthcare. Here's another factor to consider: black men working essential jobs put them on the front line of greater exposure to viruses. These jobs include bus drivers, cashiers and stockers in busy big-box stores, nursing home health aides, and law enforcement and public safety jobs.

Pandemic or not, we should guard our health by practicing healthy lifestyle habits that can improve our chances of preventing chronic medical conditions while bolstering our immune functioning.

Speaking of the immune system, boosting it to ward off illness makes sense. Yet there is much to learn about the intricacies and interconnectedness of this complex system and the immune response. That's why more research is required before we can prove there's a link between healthy habits and their influence on enhancing our immune system.[7] But that does not give us men (or anyone) a green light to neglect healthy habits. We know good health habits matter. The single best step to keeping our immune functioning strong is to live a healthy lifestyle. Doing so typically results in less illness, both acute and chronic, and improved overall health. I'll address these healthy lifestyle practices more thoroughly in other chapters of this book.

How Women Can Help Improve Men's Health

Most men who pay me a visit are usually accompanied by their wife, daughter, or girlfriend—usually after those women have convinced, bribed, or begged them to go. All doctors everywhere thank women for that.

As we've alluded to, women are much more proactive regarding their health and well-being. They often anticipate health issues and therefore are more likely to practice preventive measures to get and stay healthy. Women are usually armed and ready to fire off multiple questions, with no question going unanswered by the time they leave. Women like detail, too, and they demand—and deserve—detailed answers.

Women understand that good health doesn't just happen. It requires taking personal responsibility for your own life—unless you're that uniquely and genetically blessed soul. This includes going to annual checkups, staying up to date on immunizations, seeing a doctor when sick, and living a healthy lifestyle.

Unlike most men, women rarely hesitate to seek regular medical care when they feel it's needed, whether for a minor ache or pain or a major health issue. However, men do come see me for a medical issue they care about. Issues that, if not resolved—and quickly—can convert even the most die-hard doctor avoider. What are these issues? Any sort of problem involving prostate and sexual functioning. That's when I become their go-to guy, helping resuscitate their sex life or protecting and preserving the prostate's purpose.

This brings up an important point. Every man should have a urologist, and women need to remind them of that. At some point, most men will experience erectile dysfunction, painful urination, or some other medical issue involving the male urinary or reproductive system. Believe me, a man who can't get it up for a sexual rendezvous or is waking up three times a night to pee will beg to be taken to a urologist.

For any women reading, this is where you and I can take advantage of the situation. Once you get them in the door, I can not only address urinary issues or sexual problems but also talk about other health problems often associated with their symptoms. For instance, erectile dysfunction can point to type 2 diabetes, while clogged arteries can indicate heart disease. Even though medical issues such as diabetes or heart disease are not my specialties, I can help arrange appointments with experts in these fields of medicine to assess those conditions thoroughly. By identifying such needs for further evaluation, we can get your man the care and medical attention he deserves but just doesn't know it yet.

The concept of using urologists to assess broader health concerns for men is gaining acceptance. If a woman can't get her guy to see his primary care physician, but if he will go to a urologist when his love life is falling apart due to erectile issues or lack of libido, that's even better. Improving his health through addressing his erection concerns may be the only way to get him to make better lifestyle choices.

So, women, if a man you love is neglecting a chronic illness, has been ignoring worrisome symptoms, or hasn't had an annual checkup in years, here are pointers you can use to begin the conversation about taking care of his health:

- **Avoid making him feel guilty.** Let me repeat—do not make your man feel guilty. This is a big mistake. Guilt is a motivator for no one and is likely to make your man feel defensive. Besides, using shame to bring him to a doctor is not a great tactic for building a good relationship with his healthcare provider.

- **Avoid being controlling or nagging.** Ultimatums, nagging, or threats are another turn-off for men. This approach can backfire due to complete opposition. Also, during a doctor's visit, avoid speaking for him. Building trust with his doctor is key to an effective doctor-patient relationship. This is his visit; let him talk with his doctor to build that trust and help allay his fears.

- **Remind him how much he means to you.** Remember, honey attracts more flies than vinegar. Start the conversation by telling your man what your relationship with him means to you, and then lead into how you've been concerned about his health. Keep it positive with an emphasis on how special he is in your life. It also helps to use "I" rather than "you" statements, such as, "I'm concerned about your health," instead of "You are not taking good care of yourself."

- **Make it easy.** Schedule an appointment with a doctor you trust and who you think is a good fit. Make the time convenient for him, and go with him if he wants.

- **Be prepared.** Help him develop a list of questions he wants answered, any symptoms he is experiencing, and his medical history, including his family's medical history. Remind him to be honest with the doctor about his lifestyle habits, such as diet, exercise, sleep, smoking (cigarettes, e-cigarettes, cigars, marijuana), and consuming alcohol.

- **Remind him why he should go.** Sometimes men are reluctant to see a doctor because they don't want to take time away from their job. Remind him, though, that keeping healthy should be a top priority. Many health conditions are "silent"—high blood pressure, diabetes, high cholesterol, and prostate problems often have few if any symptoms but do require treatment. Tell your man that investing in his health by establishing a good relationship with a trusted and experienced primary care physician during his twenties, thirties, and beyond will be the most important and life-changing investment he will make. And that investment will have a huge payoff of good health, less chronic pain, less medication use, fewer doctor visits and hospitalization stays (and therefore less time off work in the long run), a longer life, and—oh, yes—great sex.

- **Use common sense.** Remind your man that delaying seeing a doctor for pain or other symptoms that indicate an advanced stage of a disease likely will make treating it more difficult, time consuming, and costly. This is where being prudent, practical, and logical can win him over to make the right decisions.

Together, let's do this. Let's get your man into the doctor's office, taking care of himself, and experiencing the best health he's had in years.

SUMMARY

- Women are primarily the best advocates for their families' health and medical decisions.

- Most men are not very proactive about taking care of their health, such as seeing a doctor for regular annual physicals or when sick.

- Men often avoid doctors as it makes them feel out of control.

- Women are key in encouraging men to get to a doctor and take better care of themselves. Certain tactics that can help them include avoiding nagging, not making them feel guilty, and assisting them in preparing to see a doctor.

CHAPTER 2

The Top Five Threats to Men's Health

Men are the stronger sex…or are they? If we're referring to physical strength, then the answer is yes. Research has shown men are at a distinct advantage in being physically stronger than women. When compared to women, men have about 40 percent more muscle mass in the upper body and 33 percent more muscle mass in the lower body, in addition to larger muscle fibers.[1] Yet when it comes to men's overall health and well-being, the figures and statistics reveal a different story. Men may be able to run faster, lift more, or push out a truck stuck in the mud, but they are more likely to be affected by certain diseases and die younger than women.

Here's what men's health really looks like, starting from before birth:

- For every 100 baby girls born, there are 115 baby boys born. Yet the male fetus is at a greater risk of miscarriage and stillbirth.

- Of newborn babies, males are 25 percent more likely to die than females.

- Baby boys make up three out of every five sudden infant death syndrome (SIDS) occurrences.[2]

- American men live sicker lives and die at a younger age than American women.

- In 1920, women lived on average one year longer than men. Today, men die on average almost five years earlier than women.

- Men die from the top ten causes of death at a higher rate than women, and they are the victims of over 92 percent of workplace deaths.

- Men are more likely to be undiagnosed with depression, and they are four times more likely to commit suicide than women.

- African American men are at a much higher risk of being the victim of a homicide—1 in 30 black men compared to 1 in 132 black women; for white men—1 in 179 compared to 1 in 495 white women.

- Men are at a higher risk of dying from heart disease, cancer, injuries, strokes, and HIV/AIDS than women.

- Men have two times the rate of hearing loss as women.

- The male hormone testosterone is linked to elevated LDL (bad cholesterol) and lower HDL (good cholesterol).

- Men appear to have a weaker immune system as they have fewer infection-fighting T cells than women.

- Women are 100 percent more likely to visit the doctor for annual examinations and preventive services than men.

- By the age of one hundred, women outnumber men eight to one.

The Biggest Health Threats Men Face

Every day, healthcare professionals who take care of men see a host of health conditions. As a urologist, I see my fair share of urinary and prostate issues. But I also see plenty of these same men with other serious health issues like heart disease, diabetes, and cancer. These conditions not only reduce men's quality of life but shorten their life span as well.

Although the life expectancy gap between men and women has been shrinking, several factors still work against men's health—particularly high rates of smoking and drinking compared to women and men's tendency to not seek help, often because they feel uncomfortable discussing their health issues.

When diagnosed early, many of the top men's health risks can be prevented or treated. That's a critical component of men's healthcare that needs to be addressed more—early diagnosis. But to convince men the why and how of taking care of themselves is not easy. That's why I want to help men help themselves. When men understand what conditions can threaten their health most, it can be a catalyst in convincing them to take action to promote and protect their health. While numerous health conditions can afflict men, let's take a look at the top five health threats we face.

1. Cardiovascular Disease

Good heart health is a friend to men of all ages. Adopting a heart-healthy lifestyle at a young age is crucial to preventing this leading cause of death in men. The latest statistics show that one out of every four male deaths is related to heart disease.[3] The term *heart disease* encompasses all the different forms of this malady—coronary heart disease, heart arrhythmias, heart failure, heart valve disease, and of course, high blood pressure, or hypertension. With so many ways the heart is under attack coupled with a man's increased risk, it's worth our time and energy keeping this vital organ strong and healthy.

At birth, our arteries are free of any obstruction blocking the flow of blood. However, throughout childhood, adolescence, and adulthood, that will change for the vast majority of us. Over the years, our daily self-care habits and genetic makeup can determine whether we will develop heart disease or not.

We know that for men, cardiovascular disease begins at an earlier age than for women. The average age of a first heart attack for men is 65.6 years compared with 72.0 for women.[4]

Heart disease has a tendency to sneak up on everyone. But it begins with the cardiovascular disease risk factors. For men, these include:

- People born with conditions predisposing them to heart disease and stroke
- Poor diet
- Lack of physical activity
- Smoking
- Uncontrolled high blood pressure
- Obesity
- High LDL, or bad cholesterol, and low HDL, or good cholesterol
- Uncontrolled diabetes
- High C-reactive protein
- Family history of heart disease, especially a father or brother diagnosed before age fifty-five or mother or sister before age sixty-five
- Older age, as heart disease increases significantly for men after age forty-five
- Ethnicity, particularly for African Americans, American Indians, and Mexican Americans

The more risk factors a man has, the more likely he will be facing a diagnosis of some form of heart disease. Many of the risk factors for cardiovascular disease will be the root cause because they lead to atherosclerosis. Atherosclerosis is the narrowing and thickening of arteries. It takes years to develop this condition, and there are usually few if any symptoms. This narrowing and thickening of the arteries is due to plaque—the deposit of fatty material in the artery walls that's composed of cholesterol and other substances.

If you could take a look inside a healthy artery, here is what you would see: a smooth inner lining that has "give" to it, or in other words, is flexible as blood flow is pumped from the heart throughout the body. But arteries damaged by atherosclerosis look different. Instead of a smooth interior lining free of plaque buildup, the artery walls are rough, likely from years of high blood pressure, bad eating habits (yep—those extra handfuls of potato chips really do add up over time!), inactivity, or any of the other risk factors for heart disease.

The roughened-up surface makes it easier for fatty components in the blood to stick to it, which creates the buildup of plaque. Over time, the plaque buildup becomes thicker and less flexible; that's why it's sometimes referred to as hardening of the arteries. Narrowed arteries force the heart to work much harder just to pump blood through these channels.

Plaque buildup sets the stage for blood clots to form. Because those artery wall surfaces are rough inside, it can create small tears along the surface. To stop bleeding from these small tears, platelets come to the rescue. Platelets are tiny blood cells that help your body form clots to stop any bleeding. If one of your blood vessels gets damaged, it sends out signals that are picked up by platelets. The platelets rush to the site of damage and form a plug, or clot, to repair the damage.

On the one hand, it's a good thing platelets prevent any further bleeding. But for artery walls already significantly narrowed by plaque, the formation of a blood clot could spell danger ahead. If the clot grows large enough or breaks loose and is traveling through the body, one of two things could happen—a stroke if the blood clot blocks blood flow to the brain, or a heart attack if a clot blocks blood flow in a coronary artery.

Ideally, heart-healthy habits start early in a man's life, when this artery damage starts to occur. But even older men who proactively take steps to prevent or reduce their risk of developing cardiovascular disease can benefit. Here are a few suggestions on what every man should do at a minimum:

- Beginning at age thirty-five, you should get your lipid levels checked every five years (total cholesterol, HDL cholesterol, LDL cholesterol, and triglycerides). Screening for lipid levels should begin at age twenty for men who smoke, have type 1 or 2 diabetes, or have a family history of heart disease.

- Control blood pressure—keep it 120/80 or less.

- Eat a heart-healthy diet (we'll get to this in detail in chapters 9 and 12).

- Reduce intake of saturated and trans fats.

- Never take up smoking, or quit if you have.

- Maintain a healthy body weight.

- Keep physically active throughout your entire life.

- Practice stress-reducing techniques.

2. Lung Cancer

Lung cancer is the leading cancer killer of both men and women in the United States and worldwide. But it is men who are diagnosed with lung cancer at a higher rate—one in fifteen men will develop lung cancer over their lifetime compared with one in seventeen women.[5] The survival rate for men with lung cancer is also lower than it is for women. Every year, more than enough men die from it to fill the Superdome in New Orleans.

Men are more likely to develop lung cancer for several reasons, starting with their jobs. Certain occupations men tend to be employed in more than women often expose them to hazards that increase their risk of developing the disease. In fact, some studies consider occupational exposures to be responsible for 13 to 29 percent of lung cancer cases in men. Common occupations linked with an increased risk of developing lung cancer include metal workers, painters, cleaners, bakers, plumbers and pipe fitters, welders, freight handlers, and construction workers.

It's probably no surprise to you, but smoking is the number one reason for men getting diagnosed with lung cancer—close to 90 percent of lung cancers in men are related to smoking, including both men who continue to smoke or are former smokers. Even men who've never smoked but were frequently exposed to secondhand smoke are vulnerable to developing this disease.

While there has been a stream of life-extending treatments for lung cancer, it remains a deadly disease and one of the most difficult to treat. Lung cancer is characterized by uncontrolled growth of abnormal cells in the lung. These abnormal cells occur in two main forms—non–small cell lung cancer and small cell lung cancer. Non–small cell lung cancer is the most common form and accounts for about 85 percent of all cases.[6] This aggressive disease begins spreading in the lungs before it has grown large enough to cause symptoms or show up on X-rays. When discovered, it is often advanced and difficult to cure, with less than half of men still alive a year later.

As stated earlier, tobacco smoking is well documented as the most common cause of lung cancer.[7] Other causes of lung cancer not linked with smoking include:

- **Radiation**—People treated with radiotherapy are at a moderately increased risk of developing lung cancer.

- **Radon**—This colorless, odorless, radioactive gas forms naturally from the decay of radioactive elements such as uranium, which is found in soil. Since soil or rock can be a source of radon, radon levels are usually highest in basements or crawl spaces of homes or buildings. According to the American Cancer Society, gas given off by radon enters buildings through cracks in floors or walls; construction joints; or gaps in foundations around pipes, wires, or pumps. Radon is a much smaller risk for lung cancer than cigarette smoking, but it's the second leading cause of lung cancer in the United States, mostly due to professions like mining in areas where soil may contain higher levels of uranium.[8]

- **Urban air pollution**—Lung cancer rates are higher in cities than in rural settings, mainly due to urban air pollution.

- **Indoor air pollution**—Certain areas of the world, such as Asia, may be at increased risk due to poorly ventilated homes where coal, wood, or other solid fuels are regularly burned.

To beat lung cancer's deadly game, knowing the signs and symptoms helps. One common sign of lung cancer is a persistent cough, especially if the cough is accompanied by blood or rust-colored phlegm. As cancer cells invade the lungs, the healthy tissue becomes irritated and sheds, which is where the blood that's coughed up comes from.

Wheezing is another sign of lung cancer. If an airway is constricted or narrowed, the air can make a wheezing or whistling sound as it moves through. If lung cancer is invading the chest wall, you'll probably also notice severe chest pain, especially with deep breathing, coughing, or laughing. Another indicator of lung cancer is a hoarse, raspy, or weak voice. If the tumor is pressing on a nerve called the recurrent laryngeal nerve, the vocal cords don't close, which changes your voice. Shortness of breath can be a sign of a blockage, such as a tumor in the lung that prevents enough air from getting into the lungs. Multiple bouts of pneumonia is also a red flag. When cancer blocks the smaller airways in the lungs, it creates a breeding ground for bacteria to multiply, which can lead to an infection like pneumonia.

The big question to ask is how can lung cancer be prevented? There are no guarantees, but lifestyle habits can help lower your risk of developing this deadly disease:

- **Stay away from tobacco.** Don't smoke, and avoid breathing in other people's smoke.

- **Avoid radon.** Test and treat your home for radon.

- **Eat a healthy diet.** Consume more fruits and vegetables, which may help protect against lung cancer.

- **Avoid carcinogens at work.** Take precautions to protect yourself from exposure to toxic chemicals.

- **Exercise regularly.** Stay active most days of the week.

3. Prostate Cancer

A large part of my career as a urologist has been spent taking care of men diagnosed with prostate cancer. This is my passion and what I do best. Every man I see with a diagnosis of prostate cancer, including his family, is always treated with the utmost care and respect. These patients become part of my family as I will continue to see them for years, even after their treatment has ended.

What every man should know about this disease is that other than skin cancer, prostate cancer is the second most commonly diagnosed cancer in men.[9] Even though the vast majority of men will not die from prostate cancer, prostate cancer screening is still important.

Screening for prostate cancer requires two things—a digital rectal exam and a blood test for prostate-specific antigen, or PSA. These screening tests will be discussed in more detail in chapter 6, along with other prostate-related issues. Men who choose to skip annual physicals are putting themselves at risk of being diagnosed at a later, less treatable stage. Most prostate cancers tend to be slow growing; however, some can be aggressive, so it's imperative you see your doctor on a regular schedule to fight it as soon as it's discovered.

Located in front of the rectum and just below the bladder surrounding the urethra, the prostate gland is responsible for keeping the male reproductive system on task. From producing prostatic fluid found in semen to expelling semen out of the body to helping create and maintain erections, this walnut-sized gland stays busy. A wise man will do what he can to protect his prostate.

4. Depression and Suicide

Everyone can get depressed at times, and some individuals may even contemplate suicide. But men are especially at risk for both. Let's start with depression. While women often pour out their emotions to others about feeling depressed, men are far more likely to suffer in silence. It's the suffering in silence that can get men in trouble. When men remain tight-lipped about their feelings or what's bothering them, any signs of depression are likely to go unnoticed. For example, we may interpret a "grumpy" or "bad-tempered" man as difficult to work with, when in actuality, he may be depressed and hurting inside, struggling to deal with major issues in his life.

Recognizing depression in men is not always easy, and it often looks different from depression in women. On top of that, different men may have different symptoms.

According to the National Institute of Mental Health, here are common symptoms associated with depression in men[10]:

- Anger, irritability, or aggressiveness
- Feeling anxious, restless, or "on the edge"
- Loss of interest in work, family, or once-pleasurable activities
- Problems with sexual desire and performance
- Feeling sad, "empty," flat, or hopeless
- Problems concentrating or remembering details
- Feeling very tired, not being able to sleep, or sleeping too much
- Overeating or not wanting to eat at all
- Thoughts of suicide or suicide attempts
- Physical aches or pains, headaches, cramps, or digestive problems
- Inability to meet work, family, or other important responsibilities
- Engaging in high-risk activities

- A need for alcohol or drugs
- Withdrawing from family and friends or becoming isolated

Not only can depression in men go unnoticed, but men often cope by making unhealthy choices—turning to alcohol or drugs or indulging in risky behavior. If not treated or diagnosed, it can have devastating consequences.

There are several reasons why depression in men is underdiagnosed. To begin with, men have a tendency to downplay symptoms of depression. Denial of depression is common among men suffering from it. But the worst thing to do is to ignore, suppress, or mask depression with unhealthy behaviors that will only worsen the negative emotions. Men are also notoriously known not to openly express their feelings.

Growing up, we as men learned to value self-control, and part of that means not openly talking to friends or family about emotional issues. We don't like to look weak or vulnerable. And most of us hate sympathy directed toward us. We prefer acting stoic and showing little emotion. But inside, we may be crying out for help.

From the time we are little boys, we are usually taught to "man up" or "be a man." This is interpreted to mean ignore what you are really feeling. The problem is that putting a lid on strong emotions for long periods of time eventually causes them to boil over, resulting in bad behaviors such as lashing out or running from uncomfortable situations by refusing to talk.

Men who suspect they have depression often would rather not know. Men already are more likely to avoid or refuse treatment for many heath conditions, let alone being told by their doctor they are depressed. For men, the stigma of depression may be considered a disgrace or a sign of failure. Or they may believe a depression diagnosis might damage their career or lose them respect with their family and friends.

This type of thinking puts men at risk for a missed or improper diagnosis. The more time that passes without a diagnosis and treatment, the greater the danger. The ultimate danger for men is thoughts of suicide or actually following through with it. Statistics show that while females are more likely than males to have suicidal thoughts and attempt suicide three times as often as males, suicide in males is four times higher than among females. In fact, male deaths represent 79 percent of all suicides in the United States. After age fifty is when male suicide rates increase the most, with the highest suicide rates among men aged seventy-five and older.[11]

Whenever a suicide happens, the loved ones left behind ask the simple question of "why?" The lingering unanswered questions may remain for years or even a lifetime. While we realize the person felt distraught or sad, it comes down to this: What was so bad that they wanted to end their life?

Survivors of suicide attempts have stated they wanted not so much to die as to stop living. The reasons behind suicide attempts are many, but in general, there are five primary reasons why men make this decision of taking their own life:

1. **Depression**—There is no doubt this is the most common reason for making this decision. You may believe that "everyone will be better off without you" or feel utterly hopeless.
   What to do—Learn the signs of depression in men. Never deny the possibility of suicidal thoughts you may be contemplating. Get help from a mental health professional right away. If you are not sure who to contact, get a recommendation from your family physician.

2. **Psychosis**—A common symptom of schizophrenia, psychosis is a mental health problem causing people to perceive or interpret differently from those around them. This could involve hallucinations of voices commanding you to kill yourself or other delusions. Because of the nature of psychosis, it is much harder to hide than depression.
   What to do—Psychosis is a treatable condition. In order to function with it, you must be treated. Getting evaluated and diagnosed by a psychiatrist, being prescribed proper medications, and attending regular visits with a mental health counselor can help if you are afflicted with this condition.

3. **Impulsivity**—Many men are known for being impulsive and risky. These same men may also make a rash and impulsive decision to end their life.
   What to do—Substance abuse is a common driver of impulsivity. You should handle it aggressively by seeing a drug/alcohol abuse center to help you face your addiction. Don't wait to get help as it could be too late to prevent a suicide attempt.

4. **A cry for help**—Men can be hard to read. You may appear to be doing fine, but inside you are crying for help. Men's tendency to bottle up emotions without any release can result in contemplating suicide to end the pain.
   What to do—It begins in childhood. Raise your boys to express what they are feeling. Know that you can still be manly while learning how to positively express your emotions. If you are a woman reading this for a man you love, practice active listening—show understanding and patience, allowing your man to feel heard and to convey his feelings without judgment.

5. **A philosophical desire to die**—In this situation, the root cause often stems from a painful situation in the past, like physical, verbal, or sexual abuse during childhood. It could also result from major financial hardships or a terminal illness that makes life look hopeless. When a person's life has become chaotic and out-of-hand, ending their life may be one way to control their destiny. The ultimate goal is often to alleviate suffering by choosing suicide to quicken the inevitable.

What to do—At the very least, you should be evaluated by a qualified mental health professional, your physician, or any religious leader you know. The goal is to help you reach a state of mind where you are at peace and understand that suicide is not the answer.

5. Type 2 Diabetes

The rate of diabetes has skyrocketed dramatically in the US and shows few signs of slowing. Currently, more than one hundred million Americans are living with prediabetes or diabetes, a disease with numerous risk factors, many related to lifestyle habits.[12] Risk factors include family history, being overweight or obese, being older, a sedentary lifestyle, and insulin resistance.

If we're honest, many of us are simply not taking good care of ourselves. Years of practicing poor lifestyle habits will increase our risk of developing prediabetes and type 2 diabetes. Even if you were the star athlete in high school or worked out religiously in college, poor food choices, lack of exercise, and weight gain has upped your risk of diabetes. And getting diagnosed with type 2 diabetes can come as quite a shock, especially when it affects your sex life.

If you're unfamiliar with diabetes, here's a quick rundown. Diabetes is a metabolic disorder that occurs when blood sugar (glucose) is too high (hyperglycemia). Glucose, which is what all carbohydrates break down into, is the primary source our body uses for energy and is necessary for our body and brain to function properly.

What lies at the heart of diabetes is the pancreas and its ability to produce a hormone called insulin. When we eat foods containing carbohydrates (all plant-based foods along with the only animal-based carbohydrate-containing foods of milk and yogurt), our body converts these carbohydrates into glucose, which enters the bloodstream so it can eventually move into the body's cells to provide energy. A hormone called insulin is required for this process to happen—without insulin's help, glucose will not be able to enter the cells.

For individuals without diabetes and whose pancreas makes sufficient amounts of insulin, there is no problem. As blood sugar or glucose levels rise after eating carbohydrates, the pancreas receives the signal to release insulin into the blood-stream. Insulin's job is to unlock the doors to our body's cells, allowing glucose to move from the bloodstream and into the cells so it can provide the energy our body can use right away or store to use later. As glucose moves from the bloodstream into the body's cells, blood glucose levels begin to lower. When we eat, what we eat, and how much we eat determines the amount of glucose and insulin in the bloodstream. When the body is working as it should, it can maintain normal blood glucose levels.

But if the pancreas is making less insulin than normal or if a person has become insulin resistant, then blood glucose levels will remain elevated. Not only will your body's cells not receive the amount of energy they need, leaving you feeling more tired than usual, but it sets the stage for serious health complications. The more sugar or glucose circulating in your bloodstream, the more damage your body will sustain. Think of this buildup of glucose circulating throughout your bloodstream as tiny shards of glass wreaking havoc on all systems of the body. There's a reason diabetes is the seventh leading cause of death in the United States. It's like a slow and insidious poison gradually causing complications of heart disease, blindness, stroke, kidney failure, neuropathy, and amputations.

Diabetes can be classified into two categories: type 1 diabetes and type 2 diabetes. Type 1 diabetes, previously called insulin-dependent diabetes mellitus or juvenile-onset diabetes, accounts for about 5 percent of all diagnosed cases of diabetes. Type 1 diabetes is considered an autoimmune disease with no clear cause. In this disease, the beta cells on the pancreas, which produce insulin, have been destroyed. All people with type 1 diabetes require insulin to control this disease.

Type 2 diabetes, previously called non-insulin-dependent diabetes mellitus or adult-onset diabetes, is far more common, accounting for about 90 to 95 percent of all diagnosed cases of diabetes. Type 2 diabetes does have a family history component as a risk factor, but lifestyle habits are a big contributor.

Here are common warning signs of diabetes:

- Frequent urination
- Excessive thirst
- Unexplained weight loss
- Extreme hunger
- Sudden vision changes
- Tingling or numbness in hands or feet
- Feeling tired or fatigued much of the time
- Dry skin

- Sores that won't heal

- Frequent infections

- Erectile dysfunction

Being aware of the warning signs of diabetes is crucial. The sooner a diagnosis is made, the better. Seeing your healthcare provider and a registered dietitian for medications and a proper meal plan, respectively, can help slow the disease's progression while reducing complications. The longer you have high blood glucose circulating in your body, the greater likelihood of damage to vital organs and a reduced quality of life.

While type 1 diabetes is not preventable, you may prevent type 2 diabetes or at least manage it more effectively with several lifestyle changes, such as the following:

- Reach and maintain a healthy body weight. Even just a 5–7 percent weight loss can have a significant impact on stabilizing blood glucose.

- Exercise for at least thirty to sixty minutes a day, at least five days a week.

- Eat a healthy, carbohydrate-controlled diet with plenty of fruit, vegetables, whole grains, low-fat dairy, nuts, seeds, legumes, and lean meat, including fish and poultry.

- Check blood sugar regularly.

- Take all diabetes prescriptions regularly.

- Learn strategies for effectively dealing with stress, and avoid common stressors as much as possible.

SUMMARY

- There are certain diseases and medical conditions men are at a higher risk of dying from and at a younger age than women.

- The five biggest threats to men's health are cardiovascular disease, lung cancer, prostate cancer, depression and suicide, and type 2 diabetes.

- Each of these medical conditions has specific warning signs and symptoms that put men at a greater risk for developing them.

- By being aware of the risk factors associated with these conditions, men can recognize whether they are at risk, and if so, they can take charge by changing lifestyle habits and regularly seeing a healthcare provider.

CHAPTER 3

Where Do Men Go from Here?

Men, we've got some work to do. We need to work on reaching the pinnacle of our best overall health and well-being. We don't want to live the rest of our lives struggling with disease and sickness, taking multiple medications with side effects, lacking energy, being overweight, and missing out on sex. It doesn't have to be that way—but it will take some work. It's called making lifestyle changes.

The Necessity of Change

Don't expect lifestyle changes to happen overnight. They rarely do. Some changes will be easy, while others will frustrate you so much you'll want to give up completely. Those are likely the ones you need to change the most! The key is not to tackle too many changes at once. Change is hard enough as is. But when it pertains to reaching a longer, healthier life, why would you not want to change?

As you read this book, reflect on what you have done before or are doing now to get and stay healthy. When all is said and done, it's the day-to-day choices you make that have the biggest influence on whether you maintain vitality as you age or develop life-shortening illnesses and disabilities, such as heart disease, diabetes, cancer, or high blood pressure.

Remember too, being healthy is not just about being disease-free or rarely getting sick. The term *healthy* also includes healthy living, as in always wearing a seatbelt or not using illicit drugs. It includes healthy relationships with others. For example, do you have regular contact with your wife, partner, children, or parents? Are you on speaking terms? Do you enjoy being around them? What about your friends? It's not necessarily the number of friends you have that's important; it's the quality of the friendships. Some people may call you their friend, but can you count on them to be there to listen or lend a hand in a dire situation? These are the type of people you want to surround yourself with—it makes life much more pleasant.

Healthy can take on many meanings. When any of us accept the challenge of making significant changes that will positively impact our health, we will eventually reap the benefits. For some of us, adopting healthy lifestyle changes will be welcomed by others. It's likely your doctor and significant other have been after you to take better care of yourself. You may have already started working on ways to reach a healthier body weight or reduce high blood pressure. If so, keep up the good work—both for you and for your loved ones, if that's what motivates you most. However, plenty of us have faced—and may continue to face—a huge challenge that prevents us from enjoying healthy living. It's called inertia.

It's easy to fall into a state of inertia. You just keep doing what you like to do even though it is harming your health. Besides, it's not easy to change ingrained habits. Maybe you haven't exercised in years or you're drinking one too many cans of soda or beer every day. You may have bought into the attitude of, "Hey, if it ain't broken, why fix it?" Then you get an unexpected diagnosis you'll have to deal with for a long time. That's why the concept of making changes before things go wrong makes sense.

Even if you already have health issues, it doesn't necessarily mean it's too late. You can work on simple changes that lead to big rewards over time. You want the big reward, right? To reach it, you have to put some strategies in place to help you take charge of your health.

Breaking Bad Habits

Once you understand the need for change and want to change, you will have jumped over a big hurdle. The next step is making it happen. Strategic planning is a must, and it begins with breaking bad habits.

Habits are formed as automatic behaviors that make our lives easier, safer, or healthier. For example, locking your doors before going to bed is a safety habit. That's a good habit. But not-so-healthy habits could be eating a bag of chips every night while watching TV or being sedentary by spending too much time in front of the computer. Forming new habits requires us to understand the reward or benefit of doing so. After all, making change takes practice and time, so we need to know the return on investment up front.

Research has shown the key to forming healthy habits is keeping the action simple and consistent. In fact, it takes about ten weeks, or sixty-six days, for any new habit to take hold.[1] Then you no longer have to think about it. It becomes effortless as you ease into a healthier lifestyle. Of course, this is easier said than done. But you have to begin somewhere. For many of us, this usually happens after some life-altering circumstance that makes us realize life is too short to be sick or unable to participate in what it has to offer. Remember, we always do whatever we feel is a priority to us. There is never a perfect time for making changes except for today. Decide what changes you're willing to prioritize regarding your health, and watch how your life will change—for the better.

Seven Strategic Steps for Building Healthier Habits

It's time to get started on breaking bad health habits. Let's start with seven small steps:

1. **Make a goal.** Decide what goal you want to work on to improve your health, no matter how small or lofty. You're more likely to succeed if you set priorities that are important and attainable to you at the moment.

2. **Ask yourself, "Why do I want this goal?"** Do you have a dream that aligns with the goal? Maybe your dream is to run a marathon, to manage blood sugar better so you can avoid taking insulin, to beat back prostate cancer, or to have more energy to play ball with your kids or grandkids. Even if you struggle coming up with a dream, don't worry. You can still succeed in moving toward your goal through these other approaches.

3. **Work on one change at a time.** Maybe you want to eat healthier, start exercising, and reduce stress. Don't try to do all these simultaneously. Focus on only one change at a time. Once that change has become routine, then focus on the next change.

4. **Make a commitment to yourself.** Writing down or telling someone of your intention solidifies your commitment. In particular, getting support from others is gold. Everyone needs a cheerleader or teammate to encourage them through rough spots. By expressing to someone you trust why this change matters to you and why you need their help, you will make your journey toward reaching your goal easier and more enlightening. Besides, it's fun to share success with others who have supported you. A few high fives and words of encouragement can spur you on even more.

5. **Know your obstacles.** Life happens. Obstacles will inevitably get in the way of making changes happen, which is why it's important to identify them.

Each day, identify roadblocks you may face. Are certain commitments taking up too much of your time? Do you lack access to workout equipment or a place to walk? Are most of the foods in your kitchen unhealthy?

6. **Prepare for handling obstacles.** After you've identified your obstacles, prepare to tear them down. For example, it's easier to eat healthy when you stock your kitchen cabinets and refrigerator with healthy foods you like. Doing so also makes you less likely to resort to fast food or highly processed foods like frozen pizza or TV dinners. Start stocking your kitchen with the basics, like lightly processed foods such as peanut butter, canned tuna, or canned salmon and fresh fruits and vegetables—all easy to make a meal with. Consider meal prepping on the weekends to prevent you from eating out too much.

7. **Reward yourself when goals are met.** All of us like a pat on the back for doing things well. Meeting a goal is no different. Maybe others won't reward you, but go ahead and reward yourself. If you met your goal of exercising for the week, for example, you deserve a reward. But treat yourself in a way that supports your efforts. In other words, deciding to take the next week off from physical activity can backfire. Instead, buy yourself new workout clothes or a fitness tracker for logging miles walked each day. Or if you've kicked your smoking habit, treat yourself to a splurge with the money you saved by not buying cigarettes.

Making SMART Goals

Making lifestyle changes requires setting goals. But they must be concrete goals. It's one thing to say, "I'm going to exercise more," but it's a whole new ballgame to set a goal with details of how you will achieve it. Goal setting empowers you to work toward establishing regular habits.[2]

The best goals come from using the SMART goal-setting method. This method brings structure and accountability to your goals and objectives. It prevents vague, unclear goals doomed to fail and instead sets you up for success. Using this method helps break down larger goals into small steps, making them more easily achievable. Here's what it looks like:

S: Specific—Write out a clear, concise goal.

M: Measurable—Make sure you track your progress.

A: Achievable—Set a goal that is challenging yet achievable.

R: Relevant—Set a goal relevant to your overall life plan.

T: Time bound—Ensure your goal has a beginning and an end.

To show you the difference between a vague goal and a SMART goal, consider these examples:

Vague goal: I will start exercising by walking more.

SMART goal: I will increase my activity by walking twenty minutes every Monday, Wednesday, and Friday after I get home from work.

Vague goal: I will start eating breakfast.

SMART goal: I will eat breakfast at 7:00 a.m. on Monday, Wednesday, and Friday.

SMART goals are very specific, outlining exactly how you will achieve them. SMART goals will help you be successful for whatever change you want to make toward a healthier life. Keep this in mind as we begin to explore some men-specific health issues in the next few chapters and concrete actions you can take to manage them or reduce your risk.

SUMMARY

- To achieve a longer, healthier, and better overall quality of life, men need to make lifestyle changes.

- Becoming healthy encompasses not only being disease-free but also living healthy and building healthy relationships with family and friends.

- Inertia, or the tendency to do nothing and make no changes, can be one of the biggest hurdles men face in achieving good health.

- Breaking bad habits and forming new, healthier habits will be necessary to make lifestyle changes.

- Setting goals, making commitments, preparing for obstacles, and rewarding yourself are some of the strategic steps needed to reach better health.

- SMART goals will hold you more accountable for success when making lifestyle changes.

PART 2

Urology Tune-Up—Checking below the Belt

CHAPTER 4

Why Men Need a Urologist

There will come a time in most men's lives when having a urologist will come in handy. But when was the last time you scheduled an appointment with a urologist? Have you ever been to a urologist? If your answers to these two questions are "never" and "no," how come? Did you know that urological health is vital to every man's well-being? Even if you're unaware of the value of seeing a urologist, you and every other man should have one. Doctors in this specialty are often a man's best bet for addressing many areas of men's health in addition to a man's "plumbing." As we touched on earlier, urologists can also provide coordinated care with other medical providers when necessary.

What Exactly Is a Urologist?

Sometimes I jokingly refer to myself as a plumber. In all due respect, when men come to see me, I get to figure out what's going wrong "below the belt."

To give you a better idea of why you need a urologist, let me explain the branch of medicine I practice. Urology is a specialty focusing on the health of the urinary tract system—so the kidneys, ureters, bladder, and urethra—of both men and women. Urologists also play a strong role in overseeing the health and functioning of the male organs and reproductive system, including the penis, testes, scrotum, and prostate. Urological health is important for men since health problems in this area are common and are likely to increase with age. We diagnose and treat a wide variety of medical conditions affecting men, including urinary incontinence, recurrent bladder infections, weak pelvic floor muscles, erectile dysfunction, benign prostatic hyperplasia, and prostate cancer.

As urologists, we also have a great deal of educational background in internal medicine, pediatrics, gynecology, and other branches of healthcare. Some urologists may choose to specialize further and narrow their focus. The wide range of subspecialties associated with urology includes:

- Pediatric urology (children's urology)
- Urologic oncology (urologic cancers such as prostate cancer)
- Renal (kidney) transplant
- Male infertility
- Calculi (urinary tract stones)
- Female urology
- Neurourology (nervous system control of genitourinary organs)

If you read the preface, you probably gathered that becoming a urologist is a lengthy process. It begins with getting a four-year college degree before applying to medical school. Once you are accepted into medical school, you must complete another four years of intense training that covers many areas of medicine, such as medical ethics, genetics, neuroscience, and biochemistry. After medical school is a urology residency, which is a minimum of five years of training in general surgery and urology training. Then, those who want to further their education can subspecialize by completing a one-year or two-year fellowship program. Like many doctors, urologists have a wide range of where they can practice, including hospitals, clinics, and private practices. Some urologists may choose to go into research so they can help find new treatments, procedures, and medications to better treat urological conditions.

The Best Age to Begin Seeing a Urologist

I'm often asked by men, "At what age should I start seeing a urologist?" A good age to begin is forty. However, any man with a medical issue or concern affecting his urinary or reproductive health should schedule an appointment with a urologist, no matter what his age.

Why the fortieth birthday? you may ask. The fortieth birthday is a milestone in a man's life—men are still young but are likely beginning to show some wear and tear from unhealthy habits. While men at this stage in life may be more worried about how to keep their hair from falling out or how to lose belly fat, seeing and establishing a regular relationship with a urologist will be one of the smartest health moves they can make.

While age may bring wisdom, it also brings quality-of-life issues. Two of the most important urological aspects of good health during this phase of life will be prostate and sexual functioning. A urologist is your go-to expert for best managing these issues, helping to guide you on what to expect, what lifestyle changes to make, and when to treat a problem.

Prostate issues can begin as early as your forties. One of the most common maladies affecting this gland is an enlarged prostate, which makes urination difficult or causes you to wake up several times a night to make bathroom trips. This is also the perfect time to discuss with your urologist when to begin screening for prostate cancer. I suggest a baseline PSA (prostate-specific antigen) test at around age forty. This blood test can determine your risk of developing prostate cancer, and depending on the baseline number, as well as your family history and other lifestyle factors, your urologist can determine how often you need the test going forward.

When it comes to men's urological health concerns, sexual functioning is always top of the list. One of the more common concerns is erectile dysfunction and the resulting declining libido, which starts as early as the late forties and early fifties for many men. The cause is not always physical, but a urologist will have vast knowledge and experience in treating these important issues affecting the quality of a man's life. We also educate men on preventing and treating sexually transmitted diseases, which can have lifelong consequences.

The health of the penis and testicles is always a concern—from priapism to Peyronie's disease of the penis to conditions affecting the testes, such as hydroceles, varicoceles, and testicular cancer. A urologist is specially trained to deal with each of these conditions. And when the time comes for you to decide you'll no longer father children, we're here to perform your vasectomy too.

Now that you know what "plumbers" like me can do for your urinary, reproductive, and sexual health, it's time to take a more detailed look at some of these common below-the-belt concerns, starting with the prostate.

SUMMARY

- Urology is a healthcare specialty focusing on the health and any conditions affecting the urinary system of both men and women.

- It has a special role in overseeing the health and functioning of the male organs and reproductive system.

- Urologists are required to undergo many years of medical training to be able to diagnose and treat patients.

- Beginning around age forty (unless needed sooner) is when a man should establish a urologist as part of his healthcare team.

- Urologists offer men the type of expertise and advice unique to men's health issues that affect their urinary, reproductive, and sexual functioning.

CHAPTER 5

Get to Know Your Prostate

Say hello to your prostate. Just how well do you know this important gland that also functions as a male reproductive organ? If you're like most men, the prostate is kind of a peculiar gland you're aware of but probably have scant knowledge about. Deep within a man's pelvic region, this muscular gland, about the size and shape of a walnut, is situated in front of the rectum and below the bladder. In fact, the word *prostate* is taken from the Greek expression meaning "one who stands before," which describes the position of the prostate gland.[1]

Weighing around three-fourths to one ounce (20 to 30 grams), the prostate surrounds the urethra, the thin tube that carries urine from the bladder and out the penis. The prostate is considered a male reproductive organ that's vital for secreting prostate fluid, one of the components of semen, making it an important part of the male reproductive system.

In most healthy males, the prostate gland is tiny at birth. Over the course of a man's lifetime, the prostate undergoes two main growth spurts. The first growth spurt occurs in boys during puberty. Fueled by the sex hormones made by the testicles, this first growth spurt doubles the size of the prostate. For reasons not completely understood, the second phase of growth begins around age twenty-five and continues during most of a man's life. By the time you reach forty, your prostate may have gone from the size of a walnut to the size of an apricot. By the time you reach sixty, it might be the size of a lemon.

What Exactly Does the Prostate Gland Do?

We know what our eyes, ears, and noses do all day. But could you describe what keeps your prostate gland busy? What kind of duties does it have, and how important are they? Let's just say for a small gland, it plays a big role in the continuation of the human race.

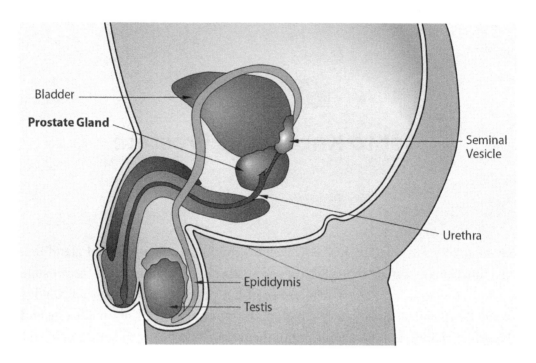

For starters, the most important function of the prostate is producing a fluid that, together with sperm cells from the testicles and fluids from other glands, makes up semen. Semen is the white bodily fluid propelled by the prostate gland's muscles into the urethra when a man ejaculates. During ejaculation, millions of sperm move from the testicles through tubes called the vas deferens into the area of the prostate. Once there, the prostate contracts, closing off the opening between the bladder and the urethra. Semen is then released into the urethra, which is the channel for it to be expelled from the body. This closing of the urethra up to the bladder prevents sperm from going the wrong way—the bladder. If sperm were to enter the bladder, it would be destroyed by the acid in urine.

The milky prostatic fluid—which contains various enzymes, zinc, and citric acid—makes up about one-third of the total volume of semen (the rest is sperm and fluid from both the seminal vesicles and a pea-sized gland called the bulbourethral gland). Because sperm need to be in an alkaline or basic environment, another fluid in semen gets involved to protect sperm from being destroyed by the acidic vaginal environment. This alkaline fluid is made by the seminal vesicles. In addition, the prostate acts as a filter by removing any potential toxic substances in the semen that would prevent sperm from doing its job.

One of the enzymes in prostatic fluid is prostate-specific antigen (PSA), a protein produced by cells in the prostate gland. PSA helps to "thin down" the semen so it stays a liquid for the entire trip and can easily swim into the fallopian tubes, where fertilization takes place. Basically, PSA increases the odds of sperm reaching their final destination of successfully fertilizing an egg. And thanks to the prostate glands' muscle power, vigorous expulsion during ejaculation ensures that the sperm travel far enough into a woman's vagina to reach the fallopian tubes.

Guess what else your prostate is in charge of? Your urine flow. That's because the prostate surrounds the urethra, the tube that carries urine out of your body. It also is in charge of stopping urine from leaving the bladder until you urinate. If the prostate becomes enlarged, this will put pressure on the urethra, which can result in annoying urination issues.

Potential Prostate Problems

As a man, there's a good chance during your lifetime you will be at risk of developing prostate issues. Every man has a prostate, and that means all the men in your life—your grandfather, father, uncle, brother, son, nephew, friends—have a chance of getting diagnosed with a prostate problem.

There are three prostate problems that should prompt men to seek a urologist's advice and expertise. They are prostatitis, benign prostatic hyperplasia (BPH), and prostate cancer (discussed in chapter 6).

Prostatitis

Affecting men of all ages, prostatitis (-*itis* meaning inflammation), or inflammation of the prostate gland, is a painful condition that more than two million men seek help for every year. This benign, or noncancerous, condition is considered either acute (occurring suddenly) or chronic (long term). Another type of prostatitis is called asymptomatic inflammatory prostatitis. This type of prostatitis is when infection-fighting cells are present but common prostatitis symptoms are absent. Men usually get diagnosed with it during an examination for other conditions, such as infertility or prostate cancer.

Both acute and chronic prostatitis are likely caused by bacteria that have entered the prostatic ducts from the rectum due to a backward flow of infected urine. Prostatitis is not contagious or considered a type of sexually transmitted disease. However, it can result from several different sexually transmitted diseases.

Even though acute or chronic prostatitis can occur at any age, there are certain conditions that put us men at a greater risk for developing it:

- Any man with recent bladder, urinary tract, or other infection elsewhere in the body
- Injury or trauma to the perineum (the area between the scrotum and the anus)
- Abnormal urinary tract anatomy
- Enlarged prostate
- Rectal intercourse
- Recent procedure involving the insertion of a urinary catheter or cystoscope

The symptoms of both acute and chronic prostatitis are generally the same even though each man may experience symptoms differently. Symptoms may include:

- Urinary frequency and/or urgency
- Burning or stinging sensation during urination
- Painful urination
- Reduced stream volume during urination
- Rectal pain and/or pressure
- Fever and chills (usually with acute prostatitis)
- Lower back pain and/or pelvic pain
- Discharge through the urethra during bowel movements
- Sexual dysfunction and/or loss of sex drive
- Throbbing sensations in the rectal and/or genital area

In order for prostatitis to be treated successfully, an accurate diagnosis is needed. There are several methods a urologist may use to diagnose it:

- Urine culture.
- Digital rectal exam (DRE). This procedure is when the doctor inserts a gloved finger into the rectum to examine the prostate gland.
- Semen culture.
- Prostate massage. Performed during a DRE, it involves the doctor inserting a gloved, lubricated finger into the rectum to "strip" or gently massage the prostate gland to drain prostate fluid into the urethra. The fluid is then examined under a microscope to detect inflammation and/or infection.

- Cystoscopy or cystourethroscopy. An examination in which a scope, a flexible tube and viewing device, is inserted through the urethra to examine the bladder and urinary tract for structural abnormalities or obstructions, such as tumors or stones.

Acute bacterial prostatitis is the least common of all types of prostatitis and can occur in men of any age. Treatment usually involves antimicrobial medication for up to two weeks. It's important for any man with acute prostatitis to take the full course of medication, even when there are no more symptoms, so antibiotic-resistant bacteria doesn't develop. You might also be advised to increase fluid intake and use pain-relieving medications. If prostatitis is severe, hospitalization may be required.

Chronic prostatitis can be divided into two different types—chronic prostatitis/chronic pelvic pain syndrome, the most common form, and chronic bacterial prostatitis, a recurrent infection of the prostate gland that is sometimes prolonged and difficult to treat. Symptoms of chronic prostatitis are similar to those of acute prostatitis but less intense. Treatment for chronic prostatitis usually involves antimicrobial medication for four to six weeks. If the infection doesn't respond to the medication, then long-term, low-dose antimicrobial medication may be prescribed. Other treatment methods might include hot baths, a heating pad, or, in rare cases, surgery on either the urethra or prostate.

Benign Prostatic Hyperplasia (BPH)

Of all medical conditions affecting the prostate gland, benign prostatic hyperplasia (BPH) is the most common. BPH becomes more prevalent as we age, with the risk increasing each year after age forty. Between the ages of fifty-one and sixty, about half of all men have BPH, and up to 90 percent of men over eighty have it.

Remember, *benign* means "not cancerous." It should be reassuring to know that BPH is not linked to prostate cancer and doesn't increase your risk of developing it, even though the symptoms of BPH and prostate cancer are similar. The word *hyperplasia* means an enlargement of an organ or tissue caused by an increase in its cell reproduction. Hyperplasia of the prostate indicates the walnut-shaped gland has grown large enough to start squeezing the urethra. That pressure affects the flow of urine and causes other associated symptoms.

Generally, BPH is considered a harmless yet nuisance condition, mainly because of the bothersome symptoms. These can include:

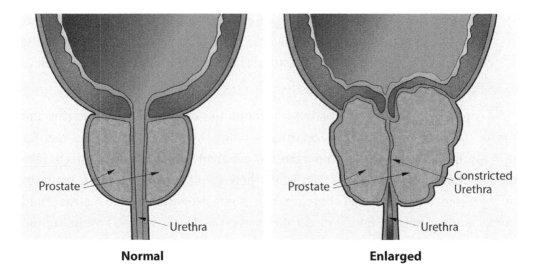

Normal   **Enlarged**

- An urgent or frequent need to urinate
- Slow flow
- Difficulty starting a urine stream
- Dribbling
- Not being able to completely empty your bladder

Probably the most annoying symptom of BPH, however, is frequent sleep interruptions to go pee. Yet not all men with BPH will experience these symptoms. Depending on which area of the prostate becomes enlarged, the urethra may or may not obstruct urinary flow.

Since the cause of BPH is not completely understood, recommending lifestyle habits for men to help reduce their risk is difficult. However, there is one for-sure "treatment" that 100 percent guarantees you will not develop BPH at any point in your lifetime—removal of the testicles before puberty. I'm very certain extremely few men (if any) would ever consider that drastic of a decision! However, this has led some researchers to believe factors related to aging and the testicles may be behind the development of BPH.[2]

What is known is that BPH is much more common in older men than younger men. The aging process leads to changes in male sex hormones, which appears to play a role in prostate enlargement. In general, male sex hormones, or androgens, affect prostate growth. The most important androgen is testosterone, which is produced in the testes over the course of a man's life, along with small amounts of the female hormone estrogen. The older a man becomes, the more the active testosterone in his blood decreases, leaving a higher amount of estrogen. Scientific studies have suggested that BPH may occur because of the higher proportion of estrogen within the prostate, which may increase the activity of substances that promote prostate cell growth.[3]

Another research theory of why BPH occurs involves a different male hormone called dihydrotestosterone (DHT). This hormone is a byproduct of testosterone—almost 10 percent of the testosterone produced by an adult each day is converted to DHT, by the testicles in men and the ovaries in women. DHT stimulates cell growth in the tissue lining the prostate gland, which is why it's the major cause of the prostate's rapid enlargement between puberty and young adulthood. This same hormone is also a prime suspect in prostate enlargement in later adulthood. Some research has indicated that even with a drop in testosterone levels, older men continue to produce and accumulate high levels of DHT in the prostate. It is speculated that this DHT accumulation may encourage prostate cells to continue to grow, as scientists have noted that men who do not produce DHT do not develop benign prostatic hyperplasia.[4]

Because of all these natural hormonal processes that play out over time, men who live a long life will likely develop BPH. Knowing that, men of any age should be asking, "Can it be prevented?" Again, there is no definitive answer of exactly how to prevent BPH. But one thing to remember is whatever is good for the heart is good for the prostate. In other words, focus on practicing heart-healthy living. Heart-healthy living involves exercising regularly and maintaining normal blood pressure and blood sugar levels, a healthy body weight, and a healthy waist size. Each of these factors will be addressed more thoroughly in chapters 9 through 12.

Since BPH can negatively influence a man's quality of life with all the urinary issues, the goal is to learn ways to effectively manage these symptoms. However, any man experiencing symptoms related to BPH should first get an accurate diagnosis. Is BPH to be blamed for all urinary problems? No, but instead of suffering in silence assuming the symptoms are due to BPH, go see your doctor. Your doctor will start by asking questions and having you describe your symptoms before doing a physical exam. This initial exam is likely to include a digital rectal exam, a urine test to rule out an infection or other conditions causing similar symptoms, a blood test that might indicate kidney problems, and a PSA blood test. The levels of PSA increase when you have an enlarged prostate, but elevated PSA levels can also be due to recent procedures, infection, surgery, or prostate cancer.

Additional testing may be necessary to help confirm an enlarged prostate and to rule out other conditions. These tests might include a urinary flow test, which measures the strength and amount of your urine flow; a postvoid residual volume test, which measures whether you can empty your bladder completely; or a twenty-four-hour voiding diary in which you record the frequency and amount of urine over the course of a day.

Once testing is completed and confirms a BPH diagnosis, you can begin practicing certain lifestyle changes to help reduce symptoms. Here are simple steps you can do at home:

- Take your time and relax when urinating.

- Empty your bladder completely each time you urinate. This will save you several trips to the bathroom. BPH can cause frequent urinary urgency, so use the restroom about every three hours even if you don't feel the need. Always urinate before leaving home and before going to bed.

- Practice "double voiding"—when it feels like you're done urinating, wait a few seconds and try again.

- Spread fluid intake throughout the day. Avoid drinking anything at least three hours before bedtime, especially beverages containing caffeine or alcohol. These are diuretics, which stimulate the kidneys to make urine. (Yes—that means your nightcap might need to become an "afternoon" cap instead!) Caffeinated beverages can also increase urgency and frequency of nighttime urination.[5]

- If possible, avoid medications (both prescription and over-the-counter meds) that can make symptoms worse. Decongestants and antihistamines can interfere with urination, while some prescriptions may aggravate BPH. These include diuretics for high blood pressure, which make you urinate more often, and some antidepressants, which can reduce urine flow. Even testosterone therapy medications including gels, implants, and injections could cause urinary issues. Have your doctor review all your medications. Adjusting dosages, changing when you take medications, or prescribing different medications can help reduce urinary symptoms.

- Reduce stress. Being tense or nervous can increase urinary frequency. Stress-relieving activities like regular exercise and yoga or meditation may help reduce your urge to urinate.

- Learn and practice Kegel exercises. Kegel exercises won't bulk you up, but they will do something just as important—strengthen the muscles that support your bladder, aka the pelvic floor pubococcygeus (PC) muscles. Strong pelvic floor muscles go a long way toward warding off urinary incontinence and reducing BPH symptoms. The exercise itself is simple, but finding the right muscles to work out is not easy. When you identify the right muscles, you will feel the contraction more in the back of the pelvic area than the front. Start by lying on your back, and pretend you are trying to avoid passing gas or trying to stop your urine stream. Hold this contraction for three to five seconds, and then relax three to five seconds. Repeat several times. When performing this contraction, do not contract your abdominal, leg, or buttock muscles or lift your pelvis. Place a hand gently on your belly to detect unwanted abdominal activity. Gradually increase the length of contractions and relaxations, working up to ten-second contractions and relaxations. Eventually try to do at least thirty to forty Kegels every day, spreading them throughout the day. Since these exercises are unnoticeable by anyone else, they can be practiced when you're driving, standing in line somewhere, or riding an elevator—no one will ever know.

- Avoid sitting too long. If you have a sedentary job like driving or an office job, or if you sit for long periods of time otherwise, get up and move more. Sitting too long in the same position can actually worsen BPH. Make it a habit to get up and move around about every twenty to thirty minutes. This not only helps stretch your legs but also gets circulation flowing.

Understanding your prostate and common ailments of it is an important part of understanding how to take care of this gland. Knowledge is power, and the more information you can gather about your prostate gland, the better prepared you will be if you ever get diagnosed with a common cancer many men will face—prostate cancer.

SUMMARY

- The prostate gland, located in a man's pelvic region and about the size and shape of a walnut, has various functions, especially with male reproduction. Some of the functions include producing fluid that makes up semen, vigorously propelling sperm during ejaculation so they will reach the fallopian tubes for fertilization, and controlling urine flow from the urethra.

- The three most common prostate issues men may have over their lifetime include prostatitis, benign prostatic hyperplasia, and prostate cancer.

- Prostatitis, or inflammation of the prostate, can be either acute or chronic, with varying symptoms.

- Benign prostatic hyperplasia, or BPH, is the most common prostate problem the majority of men will face as they get older.

- BPH is a noncancerous condition that affects urine flow and causes many related symptoms, like frequent urination.

- While not a risk factor for prostate cancer, BPH should be properly diagnosed so men can practice lifestyle tips to gain better control of their urine flow and improve their quality of life.

CHAPTER 6

Every Man's Fear—Prostate Cancer

"Your test results have come back. You have prostate cancer."

Over the course of my medical career, I've unfortunately been the bearer of bad news, speaking those words to more men than I can count. The surprise, the disappointment, the look of fear in their eyes is what I see first after delivering this devastating diagnosis. Many men who've been told they have prostate cancer say they feel betrayed—why me? Why do I have cancer? What did I do to deserve this? I thought I was healthy when all of a sudden, I was blindsided with prostate cancer—what happened?

Hearing you have prostate cancer is a major blow, no matter who you are or how old you are. A cancer diagnosis is scary, so you have a right to be scared.

However, men diagnosed with prostate cancer today have a better outlook than ever before. Early detection, improved treatments, and new medications have boosted prostate cancer's survival rate to 98 percent. In other words, nearly all men will survive it and likely die of another cause.[1]

What Is Prostate Cancer?

Like all cancers, prostate cancer is defined by an uncontrolled growth of malignant (cancerous) cells, specifically in the prostate gland. Other than skin cancer, prostate cancer is the second most common cancer found in men in the United States. Prostate cancer is the second leading cause of cancer deaths of American men, right after lung cancer. As of this writing, about one in forty-two men will die from prostate cancer.[2]

As stated earlier, the vast majority of men will survive prostate cancer, primarily because of its slow-growing nature. Some prostate cancers, however, are more aggressive and deadly, spreading outside the confines of the prostate gland.

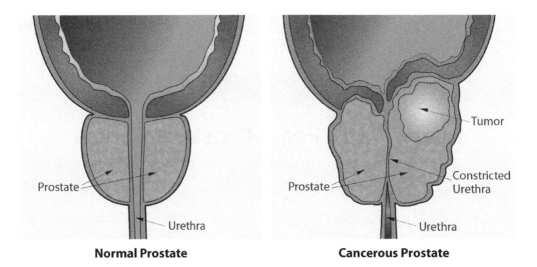

Normal Prostate   **Cancerous Prostate**

A man's survival rate significantly improves when he knows the signs and symptoms of this disease, is diagnosed early, and receives personalized treatments to beat it back.

A frequent question men and their families ask me is what is the cause of prostate cancer? At this time, we don't have a specific explanation. However, ongoing research continues to study risk factors that might contribute to prostate cells developing into cancer. And all of us hope for a cure in the near future.

Which Men Are at Risk for Prostate Cancer?

All men with a prostate are at risk for prostate cancer. But obviously, not all men will develop the disease. Like all diseases, certain risk factors predispose a man to an increased chance of his prostate cells growing out of control and leading to prostate cancer.

Risk factors are any attributable characteristic or exposure someone has that increases the likelihood of developing a disease. More risk factors will stack the deck in your favor of getting a future diagnosis of prostate cancer. But having a risk factor or even several does not mean you are doomed to develop the disease. Every day, people with few or even no factors are diagnosed with cancer.

That's why knowing and understanding risk factors for prostate cancer is not to scare you into believing it's inevitable but rather to make you aware of what you can and can't control. From there, you can make positive lifestyle changes that help reduce your risk.

Here are the risk factors every man should know to assess his probability of developing prostate cancer. Even if you have few if any of the risk factors in the table below, the risk does increase for every man as he ages.

Risk Factors for Prostate Cancer
Advanced age, especially after fifty
African American men—twice as likely as white men to develop the disease
Family history—namely a father or brother diagnosed with prostate cancer, especially at an early age
Family history of breast and ovarian cancer
High-fat diet and/or obesity
Smoking
Sedentary lifestyle

A couple of genetic risk factors to add to this list include inherited mutations for the genes BRCA1 (breast cancer type 1) or BRCA2 (breast cancer type 2) and Lynch syndrome. Studies have found that inheritable genetic changes may contribute to a man's risk of developing prostate cancer. Research suggests that men who have a close female relative, such as a mother or sister, who had breast cancer due to the inherited genetic mutations of BRCA1 or BRCA2 (especially BRCA2) may have an increased risk for prostate cancer.[3]

Men with Lynch syndrome, a condition caused by inherited gene changes, are at risk for a number of cancers, including prostate cancer.

Exposure to certain chemicals is another risk factor. A few studies have suggested a possible link between exposure to Agent Orange, a chemical used widely in the Vietnam War, and a man's increased risk for the disease.[4]

Men who smoke are also at risk. Smoking has strong ties to many types of cancer, so it's no surprise that recent studies have found a small connection between smoking and increased risk of prostate cancer.[5] Any man who currently smokes would be wise to quit.

Finally, men with a high lifetime alcohol consumption, defined as more than two drinks a day for a man sixty-five or older or more than three drinks a day for men fifty or older, were found to be at a greater risk of developing high-grade prostate cancer, an aggressive and fast-growing type with poor outcomes.[6]

Common Misconceptions about Prostate Cancer

Prostate cancer has its fair share of misconceptions. Lack of knowledge, misinformation found on the internet, and myths regarding the disease are common among men. When men are uninformed on the truth about prostate cancer, they're at a disadvantage in knowing what to look for, what to do, and who to seek out accurate advice from.

Preconceived misconceptions of prostate cancer may determine who survives and who doesn't. Here are eight misconceptions I have found as a urologist that mislead men and the ways these misconceptions can affect their health:

Misconception #1—Only old men get prostate cancer.

A common saying goes, "If a man lives long enough, he will develop prostate cancer." It is true this disease occurs mainly in older men. While 65 percent of the approximately 165,000 cases diagnosed annually are in men sixty-five and older (sixty-six is the average age), the fact remains that 35 percent of those diagnosed, or more than 57,000 each year, are diagnosed at an earlier age. And even though prostate cancer is rare in men under forty, young men (ages fifty and younger) are not invincible and can still develop prostate cancer. If prostate cancer does develop in younger men, it is often more aggressive and deadly.

Misconception #2—No symptoms means no prostate cancer.

Every man wants to believe that being symptom-free means cancer-free. Because of its asymptomatic nature, however, prostate cancer is sneaky. Not all men experience symptoms, and if they do, they can vary from man to man. Urinary-type symptoms of prostate cancer can mimic the symptoms of benign prostatic hyperplasia (BPH). To distinguish between BPH and prostate cancer, men experiencing any of the following symptoms should see their urologist as soon as possible:

- Burning or pain when urinating
- Difficulty urinating or trouble starting and stopping while urinating
- More frequent urges to urinate at night
- Loss of bladder control
- Decreased flow or velocity of urine stream
- Blood in urine or semen

- Erectile dysfunction
- Swelling in legs or pelvic area
- Numbness, pain, or stiffness in the lower back, hips, or upper thighs
- Bone pain that doesn't go away or leads to fractures

Misconception #3—Prostate cancer grows so slow I don't need to worry about it.

This misconception depends on the type of prostate cancer. Prostate cancer is often slow growing, but it can be aggressive and likely to spread, or metastasize. A biopsy of the prostate will be necessary to confirm the presence of cancer and to determine how aggressive it might be. Based on the biopsy findings, a doctor will recommend treatment based on many factors, including a patient's age and health status. Each man's prostate cancer is different. A one-size-fits-all approach is not appropriate for each case. There are several treatment options to choose from, and a doctor will base the decision on what the best outcome will be for each individual man they are treating.

Misconception #4—Prostate cancer doesn't run in my family, so it's not a concern for me.

It's true that a man's odds of a prostate cancer diagnosis double if he has a close relative such as a father or brother who had the disease. The risk further increases if the cancer was diagnosed in a family member younger than fifty-five or if it affected three or more family members.[7]

To put this into perspective, a Swedish study in which researchers reviewed medical records of over fifty-two thousand men with brothers and fathers who had prostate cancer found the following information[8]:

- Men with a brother who had prostate cancer had twice as high a risk of being diagnosed as the general population. They had about a 30 percent risk of being diagnosed before age seventy-five, compared with about 13 percent of men with no family history.

- Men with both a brother and father with prostate cancer had about three times the risk of being diagnosed as the general population, with a 48 percent chance of getting any type of prostate cancer, compared with 13 percent among other men without a family history.

- Men with both a brother and father with prostate cancer had about a 14 percent chance of getting an aggressive type of the disease by age seventy-five compared with about 5 percent among other men.

Misconception #5—Vasectomies cause prostate cancer.

At one time it was thought that a vasectomy, the procedure that sterilizes men so they can no longer impregnate women, increased a man's risk of prostate cancer. This belief has been debunked. Research says men who've had a vasectomy are not at an increased risk of developing prostate cancer, nor is a vasectomy linked with the cancer.[9] If you are contemplating a vasectomy, you should discuss any concerns—prostate or otherwise—with your doctor to decide whether the procedure is right for you.

Misconception #6—A high PSA test always means prostate cancer.

As we've mentioned, the PSA test is the leading method of screening for prostate cancer. The test measures the amount of PSA, a protein produced by both cancerous and noncancerous cells of the prostate gland. The PSA test can detect high levels of PSA—greater than 4 nanograms per milliliter, or 4 ng/mL—that may indicate the presence of prostate cancer. A PSA of 4 ng/mL of blood or less is usually considered good and suggests that a man does not have prostate cancer.

This is where it gets tricky—having a higher PSA does not automatically indicate prostate cancer. Many other factors can influence PSA, and a single test is not enough to diagnose the disease. Besides prostate cancer, other possibilities elevating PSA include an enlarged prostate gland, BPH, a urinary tract infection, prostatitis, a man's age, and even recent ejaculation. Again, talk with your doctor, consider your risk factors, and determine from there the next step.

Misconception #7—Men who go through treatment for prostate cancer always develop urinary incontinence or erectile dysfunction.

It's true that erectile dysfunction and urinary incontinence can occur after surgery and radiation treatments for prostate cancer. But it's not true for all men; it depends on a man's age and physical condition at the time of diagnosis and treatment. Men diagnosed with prostate cancer should do their homework when it comes to choosing a highly qualified and skilled doctor to be in charge of their treatment plan. Interview your doctor—ask about their outcomes for prostate cancer as well as the number of surgical procedures they have performed. You should also consider asking the questions in the following box:

Questions to Ask Your Doctor about Prostate Cancer

- How do you know I have cancer?
- What is the grade of my cancer—low, intermediate, or high?
- How advanced is my cancer—stage I, II, III, or IV?
- Are the stage and grade of cancer related?
- Is my prostate cancer hereditary?
- What treatment options do you recommend?
- What kind of side effects can I expect from my treatments?
- Is my prostate cancer curable?
- Do I need a second opinion?
- What lifestyle changes should I make to beat cancer and to prevent it from coming back?
- Is there a prostate cancer support group I can join?

Misconception #8—Sex increases the risk of prostate cancer.

I'm very happy to tell you this is completely false! Believe it or not, at one time, frequent ejaculations were linked to prostate cancer. Studies have debunked this belief by showing that men who report frequent ejaculations—up to twenty-one times a month or more—appear to have a lower risk of developing prostate cancer. Why frequent ejaculation may have this protective effect is not completely understood. One theory is that the prostate accumulates carcinogens or other harmful substances that may be eliminated during ejaculation.[10]

You've Been Diagnosed with Prostate Cancer—What Happens Now?

Hearing the news, "You have prostate cancer," will begin a journey no man expects or wants to take. Heightened feelings of fear of the unknown always accompany a cancer diagnosis. But here's what I tell my patients—ask whatever questions you want, trust and follow my advice, and begin practicing healthy lifestyle habits. Do this, and you've already begun the process of acting and thinking like a cancer survivor. It's when men feel utter despair and hopelessness that their battle with this disease is at risk. That's why I take the time necessary to truly listen to my patients without judgment. Letting them vent if needed, so they can express their worries or concerns over how this disease may affect them, is a critical component of allowing men to come to grips and prepare themselves for the fight of their life with the devil deep within them.

Before we venture much further, let's discuss the blood test used as part of the diagnostic process for prostate cancer—the PSA test. Although PSA is found mostly in semen, very small amounts are released into the bloodstream. Prostate cancer can cause more PSA to be released than normal, even though there can be other noncancer-related factors for an elevated PSA, as we discussed.

To obtain PSA, a small sample of blood is drawn from the arm and sent to a lab to measure the amount of PSA produced. To interpret the PSA number, your doctor will take into account all of your past PSA readings and compare them with any updated PSA test to look for any changes over time. If the PSA numbers are on an upward trajectory, this might indicate prostate cancer. Many factors can contribute to a man's PSA numbers rising, including age, ethnicity, and family history of prostate cancer. If the change in PSA levels over time—the PSA velocity—indicates a slow curve and a man has no family history of prostate cancer, it may not be aggressive. If the trend is showing a rapid rise or is moving fast, it may indicate the presence of cancer or an aggressive form of cancer, even if the PSA is below 4 ng/mL.

Following is a PSA chart showing what is considered normal levels, which often depends on a man's age[11]:

If you are in your . . .	Your normal PSA range should be . . .
Forties	0–2.5 ng/mL
Fifties	0–4 ng/mL
Sixties	0–4.5 ng/mL
Seventies	0–6.5 ng/mL

Source: Medicinenet.com

Like many screening tests, the PSA is not 100 percent accurate. However, it is still a necessary tool for detecting prostate cancer for all men beginning at age forty. PSA results can vary by 15 to 20 percent depending on how and when the test is administered. Here's helpful advice on getting the most accurate reading possible:

- Avoid ejaculation (sexual intercourse or masturbation) forty-eight hours before a PSA test.

- Inform your doctor of all drugs, medications, and herbal supplements you are using. Some drugs can lower a PSA reading. For example, Proscar and Avodart (used to treat an enlarged prostate) and Propecia (used to treat male hair loss) can artificially lower PSA levels. So can aspirin, statin drugs such as Lipitor or Crestor, thiazide diuretics, and the herbal supplement saw palmetto. Medications that could falsely raise PSA readings include testosterone and other hormones, statins, non-steroidal anti-inflammatory drugs (NSAIDs), and medications that control urinary problems, such as dutasteride and finasteride.

- Avoid vigorous activity for a couple of days before a PSA test. This includes activities that may stimulate or "jostle" the prostate and potentially raise PSA levels, such as bicycle riding, motorcycling, horseback riding, riding an ATV, or even riding a tractor.

- Wait at least six weeks after undergoing any of the following procedures: prostate biopsy, transurethral resection of the prostate (TURP), urethral catheter, cystoscopy, or any other procedure that involves the prostate.

- Avoid a PSA test if you have a urinary tract infection, as bacterial infections can cause PSA levels to rise temporarily. Wait at least six weeks after completing an antibiotic treatment for a urinary tract infection before a PSA test.

- Schedule the digital rectal exam before the PSA test. Although a digital rectal exam should not have an impact on PSA levels, it is a precautionary recommendation to avoid any influence it could have.

What to Expect during a Prostate Biopsy

If your PSA blood test results come back abnormal, or if your PSA has risen to a level indicating prostate cancer, or if a digital rectal exam feels suspicious, your urologist may recommend a prostate biopsy. A prostate biopsy determines whether prostate cancer is present and if so, which treatment option is appropriate for the type and stage of cancer.

Tell a man he needs a biopsy of his prostate, and you'll see a wide range of emotions. Some men react stoically, while others may display a wide-eyed look of alarm and dread. Just hearing the word "biopsy" can strike fear in most people, whether related to prostate cancer or another condition. While these procedures can seem scary and unsettling, understanding why they are done and what to expect can help put your mind at ease.

A biopsy is a type of procedure that usually involves taking a sample of body tissue to be examined under a microscope. Practically all cancers will require some sort of biopsy to confirm a diagnosis and determine what steps to take for the best treatment. A prostate biopsy takes only ten to fifteen minutes and is often done in the urologist's office.

Naturally, men have concerns over getting a biopsy, especially in such a private and intimate part of their body. As you'd probably guess, one of the biggest concerns is pain. Everyone has their own personal pain tolerance. Regardless, I reassure men they will be kept as comfortable as possible, with little if any pain.

To make the biopsy of the prostate as smooth and pain-free as possible, there are certain steps to take before, during, and after the procedure. One is for you and your doctor to discuss any medications you're taking, including aspirin and herbal supplements, and whether you have any allergies—especially to anesthesia.

Next, your doctor should review your list of medications and determine whether any could affect the procedure. Medications I advise men to stop taking seven to ten days beforehand are aspirin and anticoagulants (aka blood thinners) such as warfarin, dabigatran (Pradaxa), edoxaban (Savaysa), rivaroxaban (Xarelto), and apixaban (Eliquis). These drugs reduce the blood's ability to clot, and I will need to weigh the chance of bleeding against temporarily stopping these medications that prevent heart problems or stroke.

So, what exactly happens when you need a prostate biopsy? Here's the rundown:

- At home, do a cleansing enema before your appointment. This will flush out your colon and reduce your risk of infection.

- If your urologist has prescribed antibiotics, take them a half hour to an hour before your procedure. These can help prevent infection, although the risk is actually very low—only 1 to 3 percent.

- During the biopsy, you'll be given medicine to numb the nerves that supply your prostate. To do this, a probe will be placed in the rectum to numb the area with an injection of a local anesthetic.

- You should only feel some pressure but no sharp pain while this part of the procedure is taking place. This probe also uses sound waves to help accurately direct the numbing agent and the biopsy needle.

- After the anesthetic has been delivered, the thin, hollow, spring-loaded biopsy needle will be inserted into your prostate gland. This needle will take eight to eighteen prostate tissue samples from different areas of the prostate.

- Each time the needle is inserted and then removed, it pulls out a small amount of prostate tissue.

Aside from the traditional prostate biopsy just described, other types of prostate biopsies include:

- **Transurethral biopsy**—A long, thin tube equipped with a camera is passed through the opening (urethra) at the tip of the penis in order to access the prostate.

- **Transperineal biopsy**—This type of prostate biopsy involves making a small incision in the area of skin (perineum) between the anus and the scrotum. The doctor then inserts a biopsy needle through the cut and into the prostate to draw out a sample tissue.

- **MRI fusion biopsy**—I have been one of the first centers in New York City to use this relatively new type of biopsy. With MRI fusion biopsy, a multiparametric MRI image is taken of the prostate gland and then fused with a live ultrasound image, allowing doctors to identify suspicious areas where the needle biopsy should take a sample. This real-time, 3D image provides such clarity and precision that doctors can eliminate the need to take multiple random biopsies, which traditional prostate biopsies rely on. Even better, it has helped me and other doctors find aggressive tumors that may have otherwise been missed. MRI fusion biopsy simply provides a more accurate diagnosis that helps us identify the best type of cancer treatment for the patient without overtreating him.

After any prostate biopsy, you will be advised to drink plenty of water, avoid heavy lifting for twenty-four hours, and avoid straining during bowel movements for forty-eight hours. You may expect short-term side effects such as soreness, blood in your urine, light rectal bleeding, and blood in your semen. If at any time you experience difficulty or pain while urinating, heavy or ongoing bleeding, increasing pain, swelling, fever, or penile discharge, contact your doctor immediately.

Understanding Staging and Grading of Prostate Cancer

I'll be the first to admit, prostate cancer diagnosis can be challenging and complex. From getting sufficient tissue samples to having a well-trained pathologist interpret the results, diagnosing prostate cancer is just the beginning on the road to remission.

Once tissues samples are collected from the prostate biopsy, they are sent off to be studied under a microscope by a pathologist. The pathologist determines the diagnosis of each core sample taken and will send a written report to the urologist of the findings. If cancer is found within the samples of prostate tissue, the next step is to determine the grade and stage of the cancer. Staging of prostate cancer tells us doctors the extent of the cancer and allows us to measure disease spread within or beyond the prostate. Grading of prostate cancer uses what is called a Gleason score. Named after Dr. Donald Gleason, a pathologist who developed it in the 1960s, the Gleason score is used to determine how abnormal the cancer cells look, which helps define the cancer's aggressiveness or grade. It is important to establish the stage and grade of prostate cancer to determine how to treat it and how curable it is. Cancers with a high Gleason score are the most abnormal and are more likely to grow and spread quickly. We'll discuss the scores in a moment; all you need to know for now is that the score ranges from 2 to 10, with a lower score indicating an earlier, more manageable stage of cancer.

Stages of Prostate Cancer

The most commonly used system for stages of prostate cancer is the TNM system from the American Joint Committee on Cancer. The TNM acronym stands for the following:

- **T for** *tumor*—This notes the extent of the tumor inside the prostate and whether it has spread into nearby areas.

- **N for** *nodes*—Lymph nodes are small collections of immune cells around the body that help fight infections. This category determines whether cancer cells have spread to the nearby lymph nodes.

- **M for** *metastasis*—This category notes whether the cancer has spread to organs in other parts of the body, such as the lungs, bones, liver, or brain.

Once your doctor has determined your TNM values, along with the PSA level and Gleason score, this will determine your overall stage grouping. A stage grouping will have a value of 1 to 4, written as roman numerals I, II, III, and IV. The stages of prostate cancer and what they mean are shown in the following table:

Stage of Cancer	Description
Stage I prostate cancer	Localized cancer—i.e., found in only one part of the prostate. If PSA is less than 10 and Gleason score is 6 or less, this is likely a slow-growing cancer.
Stage II prostate cancer	Still localized but more advanced than stage I. Cells are less normal than in stage I and may grow more rapidly. Two types of stage II exist: stage II A found in only one side of the prostate, and stage II B, found in both sides of the prostate.
Stage III prostate cancer	Locally advanced cancer; has spread outside the prostate into local tissue such as that of the seminal vesicles.
Stage IV prostate cancer	Cancer has spread to distant parts of the body, such as lymph nodes, bones, or liver.

For men with stage I, II, or III prostate cancer, the goal is to cure the cancer by treating it and keeping it from returning. For men diagnosed with stage IV cancer, the goal is to improve symptoms and to prolong life as in most cases, this stage of prostate cancer is not curable.

Grading of Prostate Cancer Using the Gleason Score

The Gleason score is made up of two numbers—a primary grade and a secondary grade. The primary grade determines where the cancer is most prominent, and the secondary grade determines the second most prominent area where the cancer is found. The primary and secondary grade will each be a number ranging from 1 to 5. The grade refers to how the cancer cells look when compared to normal prostate cells. The grade of your cancer helps your doctor predict how fast the cancer may grow and spread.

Here is how the pathologist may grade prostate cancer tissue:

- If the cancerous tissue looks a lot like normal prostate tissue, a grade of 1 is assigned, and the cancer is considered the least aggressive form.

- If the cancer cells and their growth pattern look very abnormal, a grade of 5 is assigned, and the cancer is considered the most aggressive form. Grade 5 often means the cancer has metastasized (spread beyond the prostate).

- Grades 2 through 4 have features in between those extremes. Grade 3 seldom has metastases, but metastases is common with grade 4.

It's not unusual for prostate cancer tumors to have areas with different grades. That's why the primary and secondary numbers are added to come up with a Gleason score ranging from 2 to 10. The cancer has a greater chance of spreading the higher the score and the higher the grade of the tumor. Here are the scores:

- **2–4, or G1, is considered low grade with well-differentiated cells.** Here, the tumor is in an early stage, meaning it is unlikely to grow or spread to other tissues or organs for many years. If you have low-grade prostate cancer, you will likely be monitored with active surveillance and have frequent checkups that may include PSA tests, digital rectal exams, and ultrasound or other imaging, along with repeat biopsies.

- **5–7, or G2, is considered intermediate and has moderately differentiated cells.** Most prostate cancers fall into this category, making it difficult to predict their development. This tumor is in between an early stage and a more aggressive stage. Again, it usually means the cancer is unlikely to grow or spread for many years, but your doctor may recommend treatment such as surgery or radiation depending on your age and overall health. If you're treated during this intermediate stage, it gives you the best outcome possible and can add years to your life.

- **8–10, or G3, is considered high grade with poorly differentiated cells.** This means the tumor is in an advanced stage, and the cancer is considered high risk. If the cancer has not spread beyond the prostate, it is still possible to treat it successfully, usually with surgery. Sometimes radiation is necessary after surgery if prostate cancer cells have been found beyond the prostate gland.

Exploring Prostate Cancer Treatment Options

Once it's been confirmed that you have prostate cancer, you will be at a fork in the road when it comes to treatment options to choose from. My advice is to choose wisely. How you treat your prostate cancer will determine what your life will look like as the years go by. You'll discover that there are numerous treatment options available, each with its pros and cons, including side effects of one sort or another. This is why your doctor will be your most valuable asset in helping determine the best option for you. Every man is different with different needs, and there is no one solution that's ideal for every man.

Before making a decision, it's important to get input from your internist and specialists from different fields. You also should talk with friends who have been through prostate cancer, visit websites run by leading doctors and hospitals, and become as knowledgeable as possible. The goal for you and your urologist will not only be to cure the cancer but also to preserve a quality of life that will make life worth living.

Here are some variables that must be factored into the decision:

- The stage of your cancer—i.e., whether it is confined to one part of your prostate, involves your entire prostate, or has spread outside your prostate to other parts of your body

- The speed at which the cancer is growing

- Your age and overall health

- The benefits and side effects of each of the treatments

New treatment options are appearing regularly, but here are major options that doctors are currently recommending:

- Active surveillance/watchful waiting

- Surgery—open prostatectomy, laparoscopic prostatectomy, and robotic radical prostatectomy

- External beam radiation

- Radioactive seed implants (brachytherapy)

- Cryotherapy

- Hormone therapy/androgen deprivation therapy (ADT)

- CyberKnife®

- High-intensity focused ultrasound (HIFU) therapy

Let's take a look at each of these options in more detail.

Active Surveillance/Watchful Waiting

This treatment option is exactly what it says: careful follow-up exams that involve a DRE and a PSA test every three to six months and a prostate biopsy every one to two years. If your prostate cancer is very slow growing, is confined to only the prostate, and is unlikely to spread, active surveillance is a viable option. This relaxed approach may be appropriate as long as you are compliant with regular checkups and testing and can manage the stress of living with cancer in your prostate. Active surveillance means you are still an active participant in having your prostate cancer regularly screened. If the cancer changes, you will have to decide whether to consider surgery or radiation with your doctor's advice.

Pros of Active Surveillance	Cons of Active Surveillance
• No surgery • No hospitalization • No direct side effects • Modern technology and new imaging allow for more accurate monitoring	• Less proactive, wait-and-see approach • Requires follow-ups with doctor that may include PSA blood test and DRE every three to six months and a transrectal ultrasound-guided biopsy once a year • Cancer may grow and spread, which may limit treatment options or lead to further treatments • Can create psychological stress

Surgery

Prostatectomy is the gold standard for patients whose life expectancy is greater than ten years and whose cancer is contained within the prostate. It involves removing the entire prostate gland. It is a complex operation that takes place in a densely packed part of the male anatomy, but it's one that skilled surgeons do successfully every day. Its goal is to leave the patient cancer-free and restore his former lifestyle, which means sparing the nerves that control urinary and sexual function. Let's look at the three different types of surgery for prostate cancer:

- **Open prostatectomy**—This is a traditional "open" surgical procedure in which the surgeon makes an abdominal incision slightly below your navel to slightly above your pelvic bone, providing access to your abdominal cavity. Your entire prostate gland is removed along with nearby tissues and seminal vesicles. Lymph nodes may also be removed based on your PSA level, DRE, and biopsy results. If cancer cells are found in your lymph nodes during surgery, the operation may be canceled, as surgery alone will not cure you.

Pros of Open Prostatectomy	Cons of Open Prostatectomy
• Removes the cancerous prostate and can cure you of prostate cancer if surgery is performed correctly	• Hospitalization required • Catheter required for up to two weeks during recovery • Limited activity required for up to five weeks

- **Laparoscopic prostatectomy**—This is a minimally invasive procedure that follows the same principles as open surgery, but the surgeon's hands never enter your body. Several small incisions are made, and your prostate is removed by using special long medical instruments. One of these tools will have a tiny camera on the end to allow the surgeon to see inside your abdomen.

Pros of Laparoscopic Prostatectomy	Cons of Laparoscopic Prostatectomy
• Minimal blood loss • Less pain • Shorter hospital stay • Faster recovery • Removed tissue allows for accurate staging of cancer	• Increased risk of incontinence, erectile dysfunction, and bowel issues if performed by an inexperienced surgeon

- **Robotic radical prostatectomy**—First performed in Paris by Claude Abbou in 2000, this minimally invasive procedure combines the advantages of the open and laparoscopic approaches. A trained and skilled surgeon will use a computer-enhanced robotic surgical system positioned near the operating table. I personally have developed my own surgical modifications that I've called the Samadi Modified Advanced Robotic Technique, or SMART surgery. Unlike traditional prostate removal surgery that approaches the prostate from the outside in, SMART surgery accesses the prostate from the inside out. This allows me to meet my three measures of success for any patient I use this method on: total removal of prostate cancer cells, sex after prostate cancer, and urinary control after prostate surgery. What makes me able to meet these criteria is that SMART surgery is done without cutting or damaging specific areas—namely the endopelvic fascia, the urinary sphincter, and the surrounding neurovascular bundles. While it sounds complicated, trust me, it makes a big difference in your sex life. It allows me to barely touch the sexual nerves, helping preserve sexual functioning and leading to a faster recovery. When it comes time to remove the prostate gland during the procedure, these modifications keep the surrounding area as untouched as possible. Another unique aspect of this surgery is that I don't stitch the dorsal vein complex, which allows venous or blood drainage of the prostate, until the end of the procedure. This helps me control the length of the urethra, which minimizes leaking after surgery. Tiny nerve bundles are also protected by using cold scissors and clips during surgery—they're never cauterized. I've now treated over seven thousand men successfully using SMART surgery, and for those who adhere to post-surgery guidelines, over 90 percent regain urinary control, and over 70 percent have their sexual function return in one year.[12]

Pros of Robotic Radical Prostatectomy	Cons of Robotic Radical Prostatectomy
• Proven to reduce prostate cancer death rates • Lifelong 0 PSA level enjoyed by most men • Little to no blood loss • Less pain • Shorter recovery and hospital stay (one to two days) • Catheter removed in just five to seven days • Better preservation of urinary and sexual functioning	• Possible erectile and urinary side effects post-surgery when procedure is performed by a less skilled and inexperienced surgeon • Results of robotic surgery are not guaranteed as each case is different

External Beam Radiation

For this treatment, a machine outside your body targets your prostate gland with beams of radiation (X-rays or protons). Using ultrasound guidance, a high dose of radiation is delivered to the cancerous tumor. Treatment generally consists of an eight-week period of thirty-minute, Monday-through-Friday sessions.

Pros of External Beam Radiation	Cons of External Beam Radiation
• No incisions and no hospitalization • No anesthesia • Painless procedure • Unrestricted activities • Very few side effects immediately after treatment	• Increased tiredness or fatigue due to radiation • Requires frequent treatments • Can cause rectal soreness • Higher probability of developing erectile dysfunction and bladder or urinary problems that can worsen over time • Can cause bowel problems due to radiation (radiation proctitis) • No staging information after treatment

Radioactive Seed Implants (Brachytherapy)

This outpatient procedure is performed under anesthesia and takes about two hours. Your urologist injects forty to one hundred rice-sized radioactive seeds directly into your prostate, which remain in your body after they stop emitting radiation. Brachytherapy is useful if you have localized prostate cancer that has not spread. Many side effects are similar to those of external beam radiation.

Pros of Radioactive Seed Implants	Cons of Radioactive Seed Implants
• One-time procedure • Minimally invasive • No surgical risks • No hospital stays • Most of the radiation is concentrated in the prostate	• Increased tiredness or fatigue • Loss of appetite • May be forced to stay away from children and pregnant women due to the internal radiation • May be forced to strain urine in case seeds move • Can cause bowel, urinary, or erectile function issues • No staging information after treatment

Cryotherapy

Also known as cryoablation, this treatment kills prostate cancer by freezing the damaged prostate tissue. It involves using transrectal ultrasound (TRUS) to guide multiple needles directly into the prostate through the skin between the anus and scrotum. Extremely cold gases are then sent through the needles, which create ice balls that freeze and destroy the prostate. A warming catheter is inserted into the urethra to protect it from the freezing temperatures. A spinal, epidural, or general anesthesia is required. Cryotherapy can be effective if you have early stage prostate cancer, when the tumors are contained within your prostate. It is often used if radiation treatment is not successful.

Pros of Cryotherapy	Cons of Cryotherapy
• Can slow growth of prostate cancer • Can reduce symptoms	• Catheter is needed for about three weeks • Possible blood in the urine after surgery for a couple of days • Freezing can lead to pain or burning sensations in the bladder and intestines • Freezing may damage nerves near the prostate, which might increase erectile dysfunction • Trouble urinating

Hormone Therapy/Androgen Deprivation Therapy (ADT)

With ADT, the levels of male hormones (or androgens) are reduced in your body by suppressing testosterone production, since most prostate cancers depend on testosterone to fuel tumor growth.

Pros of Hormone Therapy	Cons of Hormone Therapy
• Can help stop the growth and/or spread of prostate cancer • Can shrink an enlarged prostate	• Can lead to erectile dysfunction • Can cause osteoporosis • Loss of libido • Decrease in muscle mass • Hot flashes • Breast enlargement • Decreased mental acuity • Blood in the urine • Depression

CyberKnife®

CyberKnife is a form of what's called stereotactic body radiation therapy (SBRT). It delivers high doses of radiation directly to the cancerous prostate through a robotic arm that moves around your body. Using the guidance of real-time imaging to automatically adjust to the prostate's natural movement, the CyberKnife system accurately and continuously targets the prostate during each treatment.

Pros of CyberKnife	Cons of CyberKnife
• Noninvasive and nonsurgical • No incision and no pain • No anesthesia or hospital stay • Little to no recovery time	• Takes four or five treatments • Possible mild fatigue and nausea • Temporary increase in urinary frequency • Limited history and medical data of side effects and true effectiveness

High-Intensity Focused Ultrasound (HIFU) Therapy

This alternative treatment to surgery or radiation may be an option if you have localized prostate cancer confined to the prostate. HIFU is a focal therapy technique that targets a specific area of your prostate rather than the whole gland. Its job is destroying tissue through rapid heat elevation. High-intensity sound waves target the tumor through an ultrasound probe inserted into the rectum. The probe heats to 176 degrees Fahrenheit, or 80 degrees Celsius, in a matter of seconds, using the ultrasound energy waves to kill the cancerous tissue.

Pros of HIFU	Cons of HIFU
• Noninvasive procedure • Surrounding healthy tissue is not damaged	• Possible incontinence • Urinary issues due to scarring of the prostate • Chance of erectile dysfunction • Blood in the urine • Limited information as it is a newer form of treatment

Help for Urinary Incontinence

A common occurrence after prostate cancer surgery is urinary incontinence, or the loss of the ability to control urination. It's imperative if you undergo this procedure to know what to expect with this side effect. The majority of men may experience a slight dribble or leak or may notice urine leakage after sneezing, coughing, or laughing. Even if you have not had prostate surgery, you may have urinary incontinence due to other causes such as weak or damaged bladder muscles, an overactive bladder, nerve damage, or BPH.

If you experience urinary incontinence after prostate cancer, remember that while it's unpleasant, it generally is short-lived. This temporary incontinence is the result of disruption or distress to the sphincter muscles that control the release of urine, and it's similar to stress incontinence women may experience after delivering a baby.

Since no man wants to live a life of never knowing when he may have the embarrassment and discomfort of unintentional loss of urine, the good news is there are remedies that can help you regain urinary function:

Treatments for Urinary Incontinence

- **Bladder training**—Train your bladder to delay urination by holding off for ten minutes when you feel the urge to urinate. The goal is to lengthen time between trips to the toilet to every two and a half to three hours.

- **Double voiding**—Urinate, then wait a few minutes and try again. This helps you learn to empty your bladder completely to avoid overflow incontinence.

You've Been Diagnosed with Prostate Cancer—Here Are Your Options

	Surgery Options	Nonsurgical Options
Options	• Open prostatectomy • Laparoscopic prostatectomy • Robotic-assisted laparoscopic prostatectomy	• External beam radiation • Radioactive seed implants (brachytherapy) • Cryotherapy • Hormone therapy/androgen deprivation therapy • CyberKnife • HIFU
PSA	Follow-up after surgery is very accurate and precise.	PSA bounce is a rise and fall in PSA blood level in some patients after treatment. Causes of the PSA bounce could be due to inflammation, BPH, cancer, or radiation. PSA fluctuations can cause anxiety for patients and can lead to more biopsies.
Recurrence	If prostate cancer comes back, low-dose radiation after surgery is possible to fight cancer that has returned.	Surgery after radiation is challenging if not almost impossible. Radiated tissue can become almost like cement that can attach to the rectum and surrounding tissue. This significantly increases the risk of incontinence and erectile dysfunction. Some patients may benefit from salvage radical prostatectomy for treatment of residual or recurrent after radiation.
BPH	Once the prostate is removed, men will not have to deal with or be affected by BPH.	Possible issues of hematuria (blood in the urine), urethral structures or scar formation, cystitis, and lower urinary tract symptoms such as urinary frequency.
Risk of Second Cancer	There will be no risk of a secondary prostate cancer.	In a small percentage of patients, an increased risk of rectal or bladder cancers can occur.

- **Scheduled toilet trips**—Urinate every two to four hours during the day rather than waiting until you have the urge to go.

- **Fluid and lifestyle management**—Reduce fluid consumption at least two hours before bedtime, avoid acidic foods, lose weight if necessary, and increase physical activity.

- **Kegel exercises**—Every day, practice Kegel exercises to strengthen muscles that control urination.

- **Medication**—Discuss with your doctor medications used for urinary incontinence such as anticholinergics, Myrbetriq, or alpha blockers.

- **Electrical or nerve stimulation**—This sends a mild electric current to nerves in the lower back or the pelvic muscles that are involved in urination.

- **Surgery**—If other treatments don't work, there are several surgical options for restoring urinary continence if your symptoms persist for a year or more. Discuss with your doctor if this option is right for you.

Living Life as a Prostate Cancer Survivor

Ask any cancer survivor, and they'll tell you getting the "all clear" from their doctor is both exciting and stressful. They're relieved to be finished with treatments yet worried the cancer could come back or spread.

Even though most men who've been diagnosed with prostate cancer will return to familiar things they have always enjoyed while making new lifestyle choices, they may have a nagging sense of unease that their cancer will return at some point. Every time they see their urologist for an annual PSA check or repeat biopsy, it can create high anxiety, also known as recurrence anxiety.

Recurrence anxiety associated with prostate cancer is a normal, natural fear many men may experience. The cancer process stirs up an unexpected mix of emotions that can feel unsettling. As the end of their cancer treatment nears, a man can feel elated and relieved but vulnerable and uncertain about what the future holds. What if it comes back, and if it does, will it be even more aggressive?

Living with uncertainty is never easy. The first year after surviving cancer is usually the hardest. This is when worrying over prostate cancer returning will be the most intense, and anxiety levels will be heightened over every little thing. Any ache, pain, or something out of the ordinary will cause a man to wonder whether his cancer has come back.

They say time heals everything, so it is important for men to remember that as each week, month, and year goes by with no return of cancer, the anxiety will get better.

No one, not even your doctor, can promise that your prostate cancer won't return. This may be of little consolation, but a reassuring statistic from the American Cancer Society shows that the five-year survival rate is 98 percent.[13] Those odds are hard to beat.

If you are a cancer survivor, here are some tools you can use to reduce your fear of cancer recurrence and cope when anxiety strikes:

- **Identify your triggers.** Worries over your cancer returning are often prompted or intensified by certain things—the one-year anniversary of your diagnosis, hearing of a celebrity or friend diagnosed with prostate cancer, or having to get a scan or follow-up exam, to name a few. Anxiety triggers will be different for each man, but recognizing the emotions you are feeling is better than trying to ignore or hide your fear. Talking with a spouse, friend, doctor, or support group can help you figure out the reasons behind your fear. Fear could include having to repeat cancer treatments or losing control over your destiny.

- **When anxiety strikes, have a plan.** Fear of the unknown can come out of nowhere. To avoid letting anxiety take over your life and stifle your activities, you need to have a plan to distract you when fear strikes. For example, on your one-year diagnosis anniversary, go on a trip or to a sporting event. Tell yourself you've survived one year, and you'll keep surviving year after year.

- **Don't suffer with anxiety alone.** Most men know of other men who have had prostate cancer and who very likely felt the same anxiety. These are men you can reach out to and ask how they dealt with their anxiety. Joining a prostate cancer support group can be another helpful avenue. Support groups offer the chance to share feelings and fears with others who understand. They also allow you to exchange practical information and helpful suggestions, creating a sense of belonging that helps you and other survivors feel less alone.

- **Take time to reduce stress.** Practicing stress management is a good idea for everyone but especially for cancer survivors. Reducing stress naturally reduces anxiety. When your stress and anxiety are reduced, your overall quality of life improves. Stress-reduction ideas could include spending time with family and friends, focusing on hobbies, taking walks or increasing physical activity in other ways, or watching funny movies.

- **Focus on wellness.** Sometimes a prostate cancer diagnosis can be a blessing in disguise. If good health habits were not part of your life before your diagnosis, this can be an excellent time to keep yourself well. To enhance your overall well-being, choosing health-promoting foods and exercising regularly will need to be at the top of your priorities. Other good health habits you can adopt are getting adequate sleep, losing weight if necessary, and managing stress. Not only will you feel physically and emotionally better, but you will also gain a sense of control over your life.

SUMMARY

- Prostate cancer is the uncontrolled growth of cancerous cells in the prostate gland and is the second most common cancer found in men in the United States.

- Risk factors for prostate cancer can include family history, obesity, advanced age, sedentary lifestyle, and smoking.

- There are numerous misconceptions about prostate cancer, so men should be informed of the facts.

- The PSA blood test is the leading method of screening for prostate cancer.

- Prostate biopsy is usually done if a PSA blood test comes back abnormal. This will help determine whether you have prostate cancer.

- Prostate cancer is staged and graded. Staging will determine the extent of the cancer and whether is it confined to the prostate gland or has metastasized. The Gleason score determines the grade of prostate cancer and its aggressiveness by viewing how abnormal the cancer cells appear. The stage and grade of the cancer will determine treatment and cure rate.

- There are many options for treating prostate cancer. Each has pros and cons, so you should research and discuss the best option with your doctor.

- All cancer survivors worry about their cancer returning. To reduce your fear of cancer recurrence, you can practice various coping strategies when anxiety strikes.

CHAPTER 7

When Willy Isn't Working Right (Penis Problems)

Who would guess the bellwether of looming health issues for men is their penis? Forget the heart or brain—it really begins with the health and functioning of the penis. From its ups and downs to its firmness or lack thereof, this male sexual organ is not just for gauging your sexual health. Of course, sexual functioning and bedroom performance are closely associated with and dependent on the penis. When the penis performs as expected, it's likely you have decent health. But when the male phallus is performing subpar, it's likely you have other significant health problems.

That's why from its appearance to its performance, the penis has a special ability to reveal your health and well-being. No man likes to believe his manhood might ever suffer, especially when it comes to sex. However, just like any other part of your body, the penis can be prone to ailments. That's why when penis issues are evident, you should sit up, take notice, and go see your doctor.

Understanding the Male Reproductive System

Before we dive into the numerous problems a penis may face, it's necessary you understand a few things about the male reproductive system. There is no mistaking the vast differences between the male and female reproductive systems. While a woman's reproductive system is located within her body, a man's reproductive organs all hang out—literally—at least most of them, anyway.

Visible to the naked eye are the penis, scrotum, and testicles. Although you are probably well acquainted with the look and feel of these three external structures, you may not be as familiar with the internal structures of the male reproductive system, which we'll discuss further in this chapter.

To put it as succinctly as possible, the overall functions of the male organs necessary for reproduction are:

- To produce, maintain, and transport sperm and semen
- To discharge sperm within a woman's vagina
- To produce and secrete male sex hormones[1]

While these functions may sound relatively simple, don't let that fool you. The ability of the male species to carry on the next generation is quite a feat, involving many different structures with their own individual, unique starring roles.

External Male Reproductive Structures

Just like it's a good idea to have a basic understanding of heart function so you know when things are normal and when they're not, men (and women) should have a basic understanding of the male reproductive system. Let's look first at what a man can actually see down below.

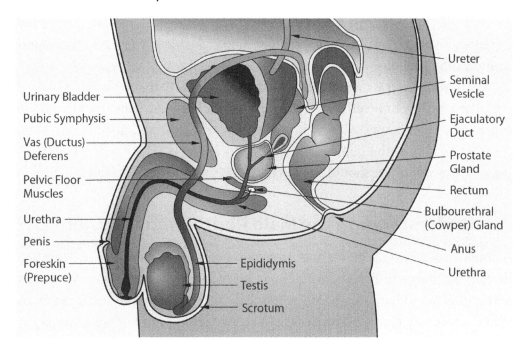

Penis

From the time a baby boy is born, the penis will be handled daily throughout a man's life. Most men are very familiar with this appendage and how sensitive it is. Intended for sexual intercourse and urinating, the organ is composed of three parts: the root, which is attached to the abdomen wall; the body, or shaft; and the cone-shaped glans, or head. The glans is covered with a loose layer of skin called foreskin unless you were circumcised as a baby. Circumcision is a surgical procedure that removes the foreskin from the head of the penis. At the tip of the penis is the urethra, a tube that carries semen and urine out of a man's body.

The body of the penis is made up of two internal chambers called the corpora cavernosa, which run the length of the penis. Each chamber is composed of a maze of spongelike erectile tissue, blood vessels, and open pockets. Each corpora cavernosum contains an artery and several veins that help blood move in and out of the penis. The urethra, the tube that urine and semen flow through, runs along the underside of them, in the spongy tissue called the corpus spongiosum.

You may believe erections start with the penis, but that's not entirely true. The spark that lights your fire really begins in your brain. When a man is sexually aroused by a thought or something he saw, felt, smelled, or heard, chemical messages from nerves send a surge of blood flow to the penis. The artery in each corpora cavernosum relaxes and opens up, allowing extra blood to flow in, while the veins do the opposite by closing up and therefore keeping the blood in the area. This extra blood flow floods the thousands of large spaces of the corpora cavernosa's erectile tissue, causing the penis to become rigid and erect. At this point, it's ready for sexual intercourse. When a man reaches sexual climax, the urethra signals the muscles at the base of the penis to relay a message for the semen to contract powerfully and quickly, every 0.8 seconds, forcing semen out of the tip of the penis.[2]

If you're worried about accidentally releasing urine during ejaculation, rest assured—when the penis is erect, the flow of urine is blocked from the urethra, allowing only semen to be ejaculated during orgasm.

Scrotum

Sitting behind the penis is this pouch-like sac that contains the testicles, aka the testes. There's a reason why our Creator designed a man to have his reproductive organs on the outside of his body—the scrotum not only protects the "crown jewels" (the testicles) but also acts as a climate-control system for them. If a guy is going to be able to make sperm and carry on the human race, the testicles must be slightly cooler than a man's body temperature. If the testes were inside a man's body, it would be too warm, and sperm production would not happen. What's really interesting, and what you've probably observed, is the scrotum can contract (tighten) and relax, which controls temperature even more precisely. In other words, if the testicles need to be warmer, the scrotum will contract by drawing closer to the body for warmth and protection. Likewise, if the testicles are getting too warm, the scrotum will relax by hanging down further away from the body to cool things off.

Testicles (Testes)

The oval-shaped testicles, or male gonads, reside within the scrotum. Each testes is the size of a very large olive—it weighs 0.35 to 0.5 ounces (10 to 15 g) and is typically 2 inches (5 cm) long, 1.2 inches (3 cm) wide, and 1 inch (2.5 cm) thick. The testicles are the primary male reproductive organs, and they have a very important job of producing gametes, or sperm, and secreting hormones, primarily testosterone. Each testis contains coiled masses of tubes called seminiferous tubules, which are responsible for producing sperm cells by a process called spermatogenesis.

The majority of men are born with two testicles. When a woman is pregnant with a baby boy, the testicles form in the baby's abdomen and will drop into the scrotum during the seventh month of gestation. In about 2 percent of males, sometimes the testicles do not drop. This situation is called undescended testicles (cryptorchidism) and usually affects only one testicle. However, in 10 percent of these cases, both testicles have not moved into their proper position within the scrotum. Undescended testicles are more likely to occur in male babies born prematurely; however, after the baby is born, the testicles will usually drop within a few months. If they don't, surgery may be required.

To keep them from bouncing around in the scrotal sac, each testicle is secured by a structure called the spermatic cord.

Epididymis

Located at the back of each testicle, this long, coiled tube has the duty of carrying and storing the sperm cells produced by the testes. When sperm are made, they are immature and incapable of fertilization. It's up to the epididymis to help mature the sperm and make it ready for release during sexual climax.

Internal Male Reproductive Structures

While the internal male reproductive structures may be hidden from view, they are just as important as the external structures we can visibly see and touch. These "accessory" organs help make your reproductive system function like clockwork. Here's a brief look at their main jobs:

- **Vas deferens**—This accessory organ transports mature sperm to the urethra to prepare for ejaculation.

- **Ejaculatory ducts**—These ducts empty into the urethra and are formed where the vas deferens and the seminal vesicles fuse.

- **Urethra**—This tube has a dual function in men—it carries urine from the bladder outside the body, and it expels or ejaculates semen when a man reaches orgasm.

- **Seminal vesicles**—These saclike pouches are attached to the vas deferens near the base of the bladder. They make a sugar-rich fluid (fructose) as an energy source for sperm to help them move. The fluid a man ejaculates at orgasm is made up primarily of fluid from the seminal vesicles.

- **Prostate gland**—This gland adds fluid to the semen, helping to nourish sperm.

- **Bulbourethral glands**—Sometimes referred to as Cowper's glands (named after anatomist William Cowper who first documented them in the late 1600s), these pea-sized glands produce a mucous-like fluid called preejaculate when a man is sexually aroused. This viscous, clear, and salty fluid neutralizes any residual acidity in the urethra, making it a more hospitable environment for sperm to travel in when exiting a man's body.

The Penis and Telltale Signs of a Man's Health

While men rely on their penis for sexual satisfaction, they can also use it as a sort of soothsayer in predicting what may be going on with their health. In other words, what goes wrong with this organ can be a way of pulling back the curtain of what's really going on with a man's overall well-being.

Penile issues are surprisingly numerous. If you've managed to get through most of your life with few or no problems, consider yourself lucky. If and when a problem shows up, you'll probably recognize it clearly. Trouble achieving an erection, a noticeable curve that didn't use to be there, or lumps and bumps seen or felt are just some of the medical conditions affecting the penis that often stem from a health malady. Let's take a look at these penile ailments, starting with probably the most dreaded ailment of all—erectile dysfunction.

Erectile Dysfunction (ED)—A Man's Worst Nightmare

Erectile dysfunction is the inability to achieve or maintain an erection sufficient for sexual intercourse. ED is a quality-of-life issue—the first time any man experiences ED can be a moment of complete humiliation and devastation. As men, we take great pride in our sexual performance. Our ability to get and maintain a rock-hard erection brings enormous satisfaction of pleasing not only our partner but also ourselves. That's why ED can be so embarrassing.

The prevalence of ED increases as men get older. In fact, age is considered the strongest variable associated with ED. Research from the Massachusetts Male Aging Study found that with each decade of life, the likelihood of ED increases: for example, approximately 50 percent of men in their fifties and 60 percent of men in their sixties will have mild and moderate ED. Some men will experience complete ED, meaning they are not able to achieve an erection at all. Complete ED affects about 5 percent of men at age forty and increases up to 15 percent of men at age seventy[3]. While advanced age can be a major factor for developing ED, medications can also interfere with a man's ability to achieve an erection. Some of these medications are listed in the following table:

Drugs That May Interfere with Erection	
Type of Drug	**Common Generic and Brand Names**
Diuretics and high blood pressure drugs	Lasix, hydrochlorothiazide, propranolol, atenolol, Aldactone
Antidepressants, anti-anxiety drugs, and antiepileptic drugs	Prozac, Zoloft, Nardil, Buspar, Valium, Ativan, Dilantin
Antihistamines	Dramamine, Benadryl, Vistaril
Non-steroidal anti-inflammatory drugs (NSAIDs)	Indocin, naproxen
Muscle relaxers	Flexeril, Norflex
Antiarrhythmics	Norpace
Parkinson's disease medications	Akineton, Cogentin, Artane, Sinemet
Prostate cancer medications	Eulexin, Lupron
Chemotherapy drugs	Myleran, Cytoxan

Source: Medlineplus.gov

Besides these listed prescribed medications, recreational drug use is another potential source of impotence. These include amphetamines, barbiturates, cocaine, marijuana, heroin, and nicotine. Excessive alcohol use can cause problems, too.

One vital requirement for a man with ED is an understanding and patient partner. Older men will often need more stimulation to get an erection and more time between erections. For anyone with ongoing ED issues, this sensitive and emotional topic can be very difficult to talk about with his partner or doctor. Yet talking is exactly what men should do. Why suffer in silence? Remaining stoic and tight-lipped will get you nowhere fast. Seeking and asking for help for a basic human need—and one of life's most sensually gratifying moments—is nothing to keep under wraps. Keeping quiet can lead to physical or psychological consequences, including stress, relationship strain, and low self-esteem.

There are two major benefits to seeking help. First, there are treatments than can improve or even resolve the situation, helping you regain your sex life. Second, it's important to figure out why you are having ED to begin with. Achieving an erection is a complex process involving many parts of the body—the brain, hormones, nerves, muscles, and blood circulation. Anything interfering with this process can result in ED, including underlying health conditions such as cardiovascular problems or diabetes. The ideal doctor to begin with for treating ED is a urologist. Urologists are specifically trained and educated in male reproductive and sexual health. When seeing a patient with ED, urologists can also review other possible underlying health maladies by going over a checklist of other health concerns. Besides, when the flag can't be raised, there's usually something wrong within the system.

Here's a look at several major health conditions that may lead to ED:

Diabetes

One of the most common and yet often neglected medical problems in men with diabetes is erectile dysfunction. More than half of men with diabetes will develop ED, and men with diabetes are three times more likely to have ED than men who do not have diabetes. Men with diabetes can also develop ED ten to fifteen years earlier than men without diabetes.[4] In fact, ED and diabetes are so closely linked that some experts believe that a man younger than age forty-five with ED could be an early indicator of diabetes.[5]

What makes diabetes and ED so intertwined? Uncontrolled high blood sugar or higher than normal blood sugar levels in men often damages blood vessels throughout the body. To get a picture of what high blood sugar is doing, think of blood sugar circulating in your bloodstream as tiny shards of glass. Over time, it can cause significant damage, roughening up the inside walls of blood vessels and making plaque formation more likely. As we touched on in chapter 2, plaque is composed of fat, cholesterol, and other substances that harden and narrow arteries. Narrowed arteries do not allow for good blood flow. This can spell disaster for men when it comes to achieving an erection—good, obstruction-free blood flow is necessary to reach the tiny vessels in the penis and make an erection hard enough for sexual intercourse.

Besides wreaking havoc on the blood system, years of uncontrolled high blood sugar from diabetes also affects the nervous system. Nerve damage caused by diabetes, also called diabetic neuropathy, can damage parts of the body such as the genitals or urinary tract. For men, this can result in nerve dysfunction in the penile shaft, eventually causing the muscles to atrophy. The smooth muscle is then replaced by scar tissue or collagen, making it difficult to achieve an erection.

Research has found that the longer a man has been diagnosed with diabetes, the more at risk he is of developing ED. One study found that in men who've had diabetes for more than ten years, 78.7 percent will have ED, and 16.4 percent will experience severe ED.[6]

If you have diabetes, it is critical that your doctor screens you regularly so you can receive appropriate treatment. Because many men are too embarrassed or ashamed to bring up the topic, doctors should ask their male patients with diabetes at every appointment if they are experiencing ED.

Heart Disease and High Blood Pressure

They say what's good for the heart is good for the penis. That's because the heart and penis have a common link when it comes to atherosclerosis, a disease that causes fat to build up in the body's arteries. As we mentioned, plaque buildup narrows the arteries and slows down blood flow. The fatty plaque in coronary arteries can restrict blood flow to the heart muscles, and if it completely closes off an artery, this will lead to a heart attack. When this same plaque builds up in the penile arteries, it blocks blood flow to the penis and causes erectile dysfunction.

Since plaque accumulates very slowly (years), symptoms may appear gradually over time. Sometimes a man may have trouble with ED, and sometimes things will work just fine. Men may notice that getting an erection within seconds like they did in their youthful days takes much longer now. Or their erections are not quite as firm as they used to be and are more difficult to sustain. Each of these symptoms can be warning signs of heart disease.

High blood pressure, or hypertension, is another symptom of heart disease, with up to 30 percent of men with hypertension complaining of ED. Hypertension and ED are also closely intertwined conditions, specifically when it comes to endothelial dysfunction.[7] Endothelial dysfunction refers to impaired functioning of the lining of blood vessels.[8]

Elevated blood pressure—especially over many years—damages the lining of blood vessels and causes arteries to harden and narrow. As you know by now, this limits blood flow, which increases the risk of ED. In addition, high blood pressure can also interfere with ejaculation and reduce sexual desire. Sometimes medications used to treat high blood pressure can have similar effects.

Research has consistently shown that ED can be a simple and effective marker of underlying cardiovascular disease that may be in its earliest stages and not yet discovered. This is due in part because of ED's significant association with impaired endothelial function, which is a marker of the inability of blood vessels to relax and an early indicator of heart disease. Other findings have shown ED to be associated with increased thickness of the carotid arteries inner layers (the arteries on either side of the neck), another indicator of atherosclerosis.[9]

Any man who mentions to his doctor that he is experiencing ED should be considered at risk for heart disease. By assessing and identifying men who are in jeopardy, together doctors with their male patients can develop a management plan to address lifestyle changes that reduce cardiovascular risk, helping men avoid serious long-term health issues.

Osteoporosis

Although osteoporosis is typically associated with and found in higher percentages among postmenopausal women, men with ED may also face the wrath of this disease. Osteoporosis is a metabolic bone disease in which your bones become brittle and porous. This can escalate your rate of bone loss and therefore increase your risk of a fracture.

Research has shown that men with ED between ages forty and fifty-nine have a 3.6 times increased risk of osteoporosis, and men sixty and older with ED have a 3.5 times increased risk compared to men without ED. The risk appears to be related to men with ED having lower naturally available free testosterone than men without ED.[10] Free or "unattached" testosterone floats around on its own in the blood and represents a small fraction of your total testosterone—about 1 to 2 percent. As an androgen, testosterone helps male features develop, such as a deeper voice, a beard, and body hair. But that's not all it may do. Androgens may also play a critical role in regulating bone formation. In fact, studies have shown men with low testosterone levels have a higher risk of fractures.[11] Men who have undergone androgen deprivation therapy have been observed to have an increased risk of osteoporosis and fractures, which points back to reduced testosterone as a reason why.

Inflammation is another reason some men are at an increased risk. Different inflammatory cytokines—signaling proteins involved in the immune system—can damage the endothelium, the one-cell-thick layer found on the inner walls lining various cavities and organs of the body, such as the penis, leading to ED. When this happens, these same cytokines may stop cells that form new bone from growing, which increases your risk of osteoporosis.

If you have ED, you should be considered at a greater risk for osteoporosis. A simple and noninvasive method to assess and evaluate your osteoporosis risk is to have a bone mineral density test. At the same time, if you have osteoporosis, you should be evaluated for ED.

Vitamin D Deficiency

Men with low levels of the "sunshine vitamin" and who want to avoid ED would be smart to pay attention to their vitamin D intake. Research has shown that men lacking in vitamin D have a significantly greater prevalence of ED. In fact, when compared with men who have optimal levels of vitamin D, men who reported ED had a 30 percent greater risk of vitamin D deficiency, while men with severe ED (they never get an erection) had an 80 percent higher risk of vitamin D deficiency. For each 10 ng/ml decrease in the active form of vitamin D, there was a 12 percent increased prevalence of ED.[12]

Why would vitamin D deficiency result in ED? One possibility points back to endothelial dysfunction, the same issue high blood pressure can cause. Low levels of vitamin D might increase ED risk by promoting endothelial dysfunction.[13] One of the characterizations of endothelial dysfunction is nitric oxide deficiency. Nitric oxide is produced in nearly every type of cell in the human body and is one of the most important molecules for blood vessel health. It's a vasodilator, meaning it relaxes the inner muscles of your blood vessels, causing the vessels to widen and increase blood flow. In order for a man to get and maintain an erection, nitric oxide has to be secreted to relax the smooth muscles so the penis can become erect. Vitamin D is believed to regulate this nitric oxide synthesis.

If you have ED, you should be screened for vitamin D levels. This is easily done with a simple blood test. If you're deficient, you can be treated with vitamin D supplementation and modest exposure to sunlight.

It's probably very apparent to you by now that if you're experiencing ED, you should be evaluated for several possible other health conditions that are strongly associated with it—specifically heart disease, hypertension, diabetes, osteoporosis, and vitamin D deficiency. This is why men who see their doctor regularly for a yearly physical can address not only any ED issues but also concerns of other potentially serious health conditions.

I mentioned earlier that you should speak up about having ED because there are several options for treating it. Take a look at some of them in this table, along with their pros and cons.

Treatment Options for Erectile Dysfunction			
Treatment	Examples	Pros	Cons
Medication	• Cialis • Viagra • Levitra • Stendra	• Each works very similar with similar results • Enhances effects of nitric oxide	• Erection takes about thirty minutes • Nasal congestion • Headache • Nausea
Hormone replacement therapy	• Topical gel • Transdermal patch • Injections • Long-acting injectable pellets	• Increases energy • Increases sex drive • Increases muscle strength • Prevents bone loss	• May enlarge the prostate • Infertility • Sleep apnea • May increase risk of stroke
Vacuum erection devices	• External pump used to achieve an erection	• Safe • Few long-term side effects	• Numbness • Absent ejaculation • Bruising, swelling of the penis • Difficulty achieving orgasm
Penile implants or penile prosthesis	• Hydraulic inflatable implant • Semi-rigid penile prosthesis	• High rate of satisfaction • Does not affect orgasm, ejaculation, or urination • Acts and feels like a normal erection	• Implants may not be covered by insurance • Possible malfunction • Possible infection

Testosterone—The "Macho Man" Hormone

Though not necessarily a major health condition like heart disease, low testosterone can also lead to ED. You first encountered this critical hormone in utero, and it's impacted your life ever since. Testosterone production starts with the pituitary gland relaying signals to the testicles to manufacture it. Women also make testosterone—though a much smaller amount than men do—via the ovaries and adrenal gland.

For men, testosterone is a potent chemical messenger directly influencing an array of physiological processes with far-reaching effects. For example, it helps regulate a healthy sex drive, bone mass, fat distribution, and muscle mass and strength. Testosterone's powerful effect also is necessary for producing red blood cells and sperm, boosting mood, and aiding in memory and cognition. Let's just say, testosterone has little time to rest.

A common concern for men is their testosterone levels. To check for adequate levels of testosterone, a blood test is necessary. There are two kinds of testosterone found in blood:

1. **Free testosterone, also known as free T**—This kind of testosterone is not chemically bound to anything else.

2. **Bound testosterone**—This type of testosterone makes up the majority of total testosterone levels. Around 98 percent of testosterone in the blood is bound to one of two proteins—albumin or sex hormone binding globulin (SHBG).

Your doctor will look at both free and bound testosterone and total the levels. With testosterone, the levels will vary throughout the day, with the highest levels in the morning and lower levels in the evening. For the most reliable results, testosterone is typically checked early in the morning, before 10 a.m., when levels are highest due to your circadian rhythm (also known as your sleep/wake cycle or body clock), a natural, internal time clock designed to regulate feelings of sleepiness and wakefulness over a 24-hour period.[14] This is why humans are most alert during the day due to daylight and are ready to fall asleep when it turns dark in the evening.

Here are the general values for a male age nineteen or older[15]:

- Testosterone total should be 300–950 ng/dL
- Free testosterone should be 9–30 ng/dL

If you haven't had your testosterone levels checked recently, you should see your doctor if you have any of these telltale signs of low testosterone:

Signs and Symptoms of Low Testosterone in Men

Low sex drive or libido

Weaker and fewer erections

Decrease in muscle mass and strength

Thinning bones or osteoporosis

Increase in central body fat

Difficulty concentrating or poor memory

Feeling depressed or decrease in self-confidence

Low energy

Difficulty sleeping

Enlargement of breasts, or gynecomastia

If your tests reveal you have a low testosterone level, you may need testosterone replacement therapy (TRT). TRT is a class of hormone replacement therapy in which testosterone is being replaced to counter the effects of male hypogonadism, a condition in which the testicles are not working properly. Aside from low testosterone, hypogonadism is accompanied by symptoms like low energy and low sexual desire.

As mentioned in the ED treatment options table (page 89), there are several different delivery options for TRT, including injections, patches, gels, and implantable pellets, each with their own advantages and disadvantages. A physician will determine which option is best for you, keeping in mind that the goal of TRT is to help men with hypogonadism achieve the highest quality of life, reduce disability, and add life to their years.

Benefits of Testosterone Replacement Therapy

TRT helps restore hormone levels to the normal range by mimicking the natural production of testosterone, alleviating symptoms of low testosterone without significant side effects or safety concerns.

The benefits of TRT may include:

- Improved sexual desire and functioning
- Improved bone mineral density
- Improved muscle mass and strength

- Improved mood, energy, and quality of life
- Improved cognitive function
- Improved blood pressure, type 2 diabetes, and cardiovascular disease

Risks of Testosterone Replacement Therapy

To avoid unnecessary risks, not all men should take TRT, and if they do, it should only be administered under a medical doctor's supervision. TRT is not a substitute for taking care of yourself. If you have multiple medical issues, taking TRT will not magically cure you of your ills.

While TRT may be the fountain of youth for some men, there are also risks associated with it. These risks depend on your age, life circumstances, and medical conditions. They may include:

- Stimulating growth and aggravating symptoms in men with locally advanced and metastatic prostate cancer (men with prostate cancer should never use TRT without consulting with their doctor)
- Worsening signs and symptoms of an enlarged prostate or BPH
- Suppressing fertility by reducing sperm production
- Worsening sleep apnea symptoms
- Increasing the risk of blood clots
- Problems with administrating TRT itself

Priapism—An Erection That Won't Go Away

If erectile dysfunction is a penis that won't work, priapism is just the opposite. Priapism is a condition that affects the penis by causing a prolonged erection. While this may sound like a dream come true, any man who has experienced this phenomenon will not want a repeat performance.

Priapism was named for Priapus, the Greek god of fertility who sported an oversized, eternally erect penis. Trust me, a permanently rigid penis is not what any man should wish for. Priapism is an excruciatingly painful condition in which a man has an abnormal erection due to blood that has engorged the penis and is failing to drain out.

Believe it or not, every year, emergency rooms across the nation see thousands of men with this distressing condition. When does a man know it's time for medical intervention? You've probably heard the answer in ED drug commercials—if an erection lasts at least four hours and isn't going down or is causing tremendous pain. And yes, priapism is considered an emergency—it can result in permanent damage to the penis and affect a man's ability to ever have an erection again. If that doesn't get a man to see a doctor, I don't know what will.

Priapism can be categorized into two types—ischemic priapism and nonischemic priapism. Ischemic priapism, the most common form, occurs when blood is not able to flow back out of the penis. Symptoms include the following:

- An erection lasting more than four hours not due to sexual stimulation

- The penile shaft is very rigid, but the glans or tip of the penis is soft

- The pain becomes progressively worse with time

One cause of ischemic priapism is sickle cell anemia. This is an inherited disorder known for its crescent-moon-shaped red blood cells (hence the name "sickle" cells) that become rigid and sticky. With this form of anemia, there are not enough healthy red blood cells to carry adequate oxygen throughout the body. These cells can block the blood vessels in the penis, preventing blood from flowing back out of an erect penis. Other causes can include leukemia, multiple myeloma, and non-Hodgkin's lymphoma. Prescription medications are also associated with ischemic priapism, such as ED medications (though considered rare), antidepressants, blood thinners, testosterone therapy, and ADHD medications.

Ischemic priapism can lead to complications. When the penis is erect for more than four hours, blood trapped in the penis will be deprived of oxygen. When blood can't circulate and carry oxygen to the cells that make up the structure of the penis, those cells start to die. This can result in tissue damage, scar tissue, and, in extreme cases if not treated, permanent erectile dysfunction.

Nonischemic priapism, the second type of priapism, can occur when penile blood flow is not regulated normally. It's usually painless. The symptoms of this type include:

- Erection lasting more than four hours that is not due to sexual stimulation

- The penis is erect but not as rigid as in ischemic priapism

Again, a visit to the emergency room is necessary for any man whose erection lasts more than four hours or who is in extreme pain. At the ER, a doctor will determine if the prolonged erection is due to ischemic or nonischemic priapism, as each type has its own specific treatment.

If priapism is considered ischemic, there are several ways to treat it:

- The excess blood can be drained from the penis using a small needle and syringe. This helps relieve pain by removing oxygen-poor blood.

- A sympathomimetic drug (which affects the sympathetic, or involuntary, nervous system) may be injected into the penis, constricting blood vessels that are carrying blood into the penis.

- Surgery may be performed if other treatments do not help. This would involve rerouting blood flow so the blood flows into the penis normally.

Nonischemic priapism usually goes away on its own without treatment. This type of priapism does not cause any risk to the penis like ischemic priapism does. However, a possible treatment could be putting ice packs and pressure on your perineum, which is found between the base of the penis and the anus, to stop the erection.

Peyronie's Disease—When Things Are Not Looking Very Straight

If there is one area of the body men scrutinize the most, it's their penis. From its length to its thickness, men usually know this organ very well. Men also know that typically, an erect penis should be saluting straight ahead. Any change in appearance likely will get their attention, like a slight curve or the penis leaning to the left or right. In fact, each of these examples could be a sign of Peyronie's disease.

Peyronie's disease is when scar tissue or plaque forms in the penis. Men past the age of forty are at a greater risk, as it affects 1 to 23 percent of men ages forty to seventy. Younger men are rarely affected.

Scar tissue or plaque that forms in Peyronie's disease is not the same type of plaque that develops in a person's arteries, so it's not associated with heart disease. Peyronie's is considered noncancerous and noncontagious, and it's not caused by a sexually transmitted disease. Instead, this plaque builds up inside the tissues of a thick, elastic membrane called the tunica albuginea, usually seen in either the top or bottom of the penis.

Symptoms of Peyronie's disease can range from mild to severe, and they can develop either slowly or suddenly. Here are typical symptoms most men will have:

- A curve in the penis when it is erect—usually upward

- A thickened area or hard lump (plaque) in the shaft of the penis

- Painful erections and sexual intercourse

- A misshapen look to the penis, like an hourglass

- Loss of length or girth of the penis
- Erectile dysfunction

Why would a man develop Peyronie's disease? While the condition is not completely understood, some possible reasons could be aging, a family history, chronic or repeated injury to the penis, an autoimmune disease that attacks certain areas of the body's cells and organs, or an injury to the penis, such as being bent during sex. Be careful with vigorous sex—in addition to contributing to this disease, it can cause microscopic tears in the penis.

If you notice a change in the appearance of your penis, you need to see your doctor right away. Don't wait, as your chances for serious complications can increase. These complications include erectile dysfunction, anxiety and stress, and difficulty having kids.

Peyronie's disease can be treated depending on how severe the condition is (another reason to see a urologist right away). Nonsurgical treatment options include medications and steroid injections into the affected area. If medication isn't effective, then surgery will be the next best option. The Nesbit plication surgery is a very good treatment for penile curvature of Peyronie's disease. It straightens the curve by shortening the long side of the erect penis. Good candidates include men who are in the mature phase of the disease, can still maintain an erection, and have a penile curve that significantly interferes with sexual intercourse—meaning the angle of the bend is so severe that it completely prevents or compromises penetration, causing discomfort to either partner during penetration.

Premature Ejaculation—A Quick Look at a Common Problem

Timing is everything when it comes to sex. Sexual satisfaction relies on enough time for foreplay, time for actual penetration, and time for sensuous and erotic afterplay. But if you reach orgasm much sooner than your partner and disrupt the sexual sequences, it can feel more like a "wham, bam, thank you, ma'am" moment.

Men who routinely ejaculate prematurely during sex experience a great deal of frustration—for themselves and their partner. It's estimated that as many as one out of every three men experience it at some time in their lives. In fact, across all age groups, premature ejaculation rivals erectile dysfunction as a common sexual complaint among men, and it's the most common sexual dysfunction in men under forty.[16]

For you to be diagnosed with premature ejaculation, you must meet certain criteria: always or nearly always ejaculating within one minute of penetration;

inability to delay ejaculation during intercourse all or nearly all the time; and distress and frustration to the point of avoiding sexual intimacy.[17]

The exact cause of premature ejaculation is unknown, but both psychological and biological factors contribute to the problem. Psychological contributors include feeling rushed to reach climax in different situations or feeling guilty and hastening sexual encounters. These feelings can linger to where a man is experiencing them often. Anxiety also plays a role, especially if you're anxious about maintaining an erection or worried about sexual performance or relationship issues.

Biological factors could also come into play, including abnormal hormonal levels, thyroid problems, inherited traits, inflammation and infection of the prostate or urethra, or abnormal reflex activity of the ejaculatory system.

Whether men actually bring up problems of premature ejaculation with their doctor depends on their comfort level discussing it. I've said it before, though—this is exactly what men with premature ejaculation should do. Finding out whether it's treatable can improve your sex life immensely. With some time and effort, it can be remedied, starting with simple behavioral techniques. These techniques might include masturbating an hour or two before intercourse to help delay ejaculation during sex. Another trick is to take a few days off from sex and instead focus on sexual play, with no pressure to have intercourse.

Probably one of the most unique behavioral techniques stems from the highly renowned sex therapists, Masters and Johnson, who pioneered research and made great strides in sex and sexual dysfunction during the 1950s and 1960s. Their suggestion for premature ejaculation is called the squeeze-pause method.

Squeeze-Pause Method for Premature Ejaculation

- Couple engages in sexual foreplay or direct stimulation of the penis.
- Once an orgasm is imminent, all stimulation to the penis stops. Either the man pulls out of the vagina or masturbation should cease.
- The man grips and squeezes the penis at the top of the shaft just below the head or glans. He applies pressure to this area with his thumb and forefinger/middle finger to stop ejaculation and continues this until the feeling of an orgasm subsides.
- The man repeats this process each time he feels like he will climax. This can be repeated as often as desired to delay ejaculation, helping lengthen the total time engaged in sexual activity.

Using the squeeze-pause method can help you train your body to recognize when orgasm is about to happen so you can better understand and control how to delay ejaculation. Eventually, with enough practice, you and your partner can enjoy a pleasurable sex life without worrying over premature ejaculation.

Other common treatments include using condoms to reduce penis sensitivity and therefore delay ejaculation, or relying on anesthetic creams and sprays such as benzocaine, lidocaine, or prilocaine. When applied to the penis ten to fifteen minutes before sex, these numbing agents reduce sensation and help delay ejaculation. Even some oral medications can delay orgasm. However, none of them are approved by the FDA to treat premature ejaculation, so you should have a thorough discussion with your doctor before using any of them. These medications include antidepressants such as Lexapro, Zoloft, and Prozac; analgesics such as tramadol and phosphodiesterase-5 inhibitors; and the same medications used to treat erectile dysfunction, such as Viagra, Cialis, and Levitra.

Penile Cancer—Be Alert to This Rare Disease

Penile cancer, or cancer of the penis, is a rare condition, with fewer than twenty thousand cases in the United States, or about one in one hundred thousand men. In other parts of the world, namely Asia, South America, and Africa, it can account for up to 10 percent of cancers found in men.[18]

Finding it early is critical before it becomes disfiguring or life-threatening. Since men see and touch their penis every day when urinating or taking a shower, this provides an opportunity to catch penile cancer early by doing a quick check for symptoms on the foreskin, shaft, or head of their penis. If you discover any of the following changes, you should see your doctor right away:

- An area of skin becoming thicker and/or changing color
- A lump on the penis
- An ulcer (sore) that might bleed
- A reddish, velvety rash
- Small, crusty bumps
- Flat, bluish-brown growths
- Smelly discharge (fluid) under the foreskin
- Swelling

Just because a man has symptoms does not automatically mean he has penile cancer. It's possible the symptoms are from a bacterial or fungal infection, or even an allergic reaction. But ignoring symptoms can become deadly. Delaying a diagnosis only provides an opportunity for the cancer to advance to a more difficult-to-treat stage. Unfortunately, many men don't seek medical help because they're embarrassed of showing their doctor or afraid of treatment such as surgery. I can't express enough that the sooner you seek help, the better chance you have of beating penile cancer.

The cause of penile cancer is not known, but certain risk factors increase the chances of getting it, including:

- Age—Penile cancer rarely affects men under forty and is most common in men sixty and older.
- Human papilloma virus (HPV)—About half of all men with penile cancer also have HPV, according to the American Cancer Society.
- Smoking—Chemicals found in cigarettes can damage cells in the penis, increasing the risk of penile cancer.
- AIDS—Men with AIDS are more likely to smoke and have HPV, risk factors for penile cancer.
- Uncircumcised men—Circumcision reduces the risk of developing HPV.
- Phimosis—With this condition, the foreskin becomes too tight to be pulled back over the head of the penis in men who are uncircumcised. If the underneath portion of the foreskin is difficult to keep clean, a buildup of a thick, smelly substance called smegma can develop. Smegma does not directly cause penile cancer, but it can irritate and inflame the penis, possibly increasing the risk.
- Poor hygiene.
- Multiple sex partners.

Diagnosing penile cancer is done with a physical exam and biopsy. If cancer is detected, doctors will use imaging tests, including CT scans, MRIs, or ultrasounds, to determine the cancer's stage. Surgery is the most common treatment and may involve laser surgery, circumcision, removing part or all of the penis, and sometimes removing lymph nodes in the groin. Radiation and chemotherapy are also common treatments, often in combination with surgery. Depending on the stage and the patient, immunotherapy, a type of biological therapy using natural or artificial substances to change the way cells behave, may also be used.

Testicular Cancer—A Young Man's Disease

Testicular cancer is another rare cancer found in men. About one in every 250 men in the United States will develop cancer within the testes at some point during their lifetime, with young men being at the greatest risk. Most cases occur in men ages fifteen to thirty-nine, with an average diagnosis age of thirty-three. Only 9 percent of men with testicular cancer are older than fifty.

Testicular cancer develops when abnormal cells begin to grow uncontrollably in the testes. Possible risk factors include:

- Caucasian men, who are five to ten times more likely to get it than African American men, especially if it has spread to the lymph nodes when diagnosed[19]

- Asian American, Latino, and Native American men, who also have higher rates than African American men

- Cryptorchidism

- Family history of testicular cancer

- HIV

- Klinefelter's syndrome, a genetic condition causing underdeveloped testicles

- A previous diagnosis of testicular cancer

The most common symptom of this cancer is swelling or a painless lump in a testicle, with some lumps being as small as a pea. Swelling may feel like an irregular thickening. Additional symptoms might include:

- An ache or pain in the back, groin, lower abdomen, or scrotum

- A change in the usual size or feel of the testicle

- A sensation of heaviness in the scrotum or bloating in the lower abdomen

Any change within the testicles needs a doctor's evaluation right away. The sooner it's caught, the better the chance of survival and a full recovery.

To diagnose testicular cancer, a physician will physically examine the testicles, order blood tests to measure certain proteins and enzymes released by cancerous tumors, and order ultrasound scans that help locate and determine the size of the tumor.

If the tumor is cancerous, the first treatment is usually surgery to remove the testicle. The remaining testicle—nearly 99 percent of men have cancer in only one testicle—has the ability to produce enough hormones to maintain a man's beard, sex drive, deep voice, and other masculine features.

After surgery, chemotherapy or radiation therapy may be recommended. Men should discuss with their doctor any ramifications from treatment, such as fertility side effects.

Just like women are encouraged to do monthly breast self-exams, all men should do monthly testicular self-exams so they can become familiar with what feels and looks normal.[20]

Balanitis—An Infection in a Sensitive Area

Balanitis is an inflammation/infection of the glans (head) of the penis, one of the most sensitive areas of this male organ. If the foreskin is also inflamed, the condition is called balanoposthitis.

Balanitis is more likely to occur if you have not been circumcised and can happen at any age. If you have been circumcised, you're unlikely to develop it. Symptoms of this infection include penile pain, swelling and itching, a rash on the penis, and a strong-smelling discharge from the penis.

The most common cause of balanitis is poor hygiene in uncircumcised males.[21] Men with diabetes who are uncircumcised have a high (35 percent) prevalence of balanitis.[22] Circumcision is surgery that removes the retractable skin covering the tip of the penis, known as the foreskin (if the penis is the banana, the foreskin is the peel). Removing the foreskin makes it easier to wash the penis; however, boys with uncircumcised penises can be taught to wash regularly beneath the foreskin.

If this area of the penis on an uncircumcised male is not properly cleaned, bacteria, sweat, dead skin cells, and debris can build up around the glans and lead to inflammation. Other causes of balanitis include dermatitis and infection from a yeast infection or sexually transmitted disease.

Fortunately, balanitis is easily treated. If you think you have balanitis, you should first see your doctor just to rule out a sexually transmitted disease. Treatment for balanitis includes good hygiene along with an antibiotic or antifungal medication. But if balanitis is severe or frequently recurring, circumcision may be the best treatment.

Bump, Lumps, or Sores on the Penis—Could It Be an STD?

Sexually transmitted diseases (STDs) are infections spread by sexual contact. For men, these infections are typically passed from person to person through vaginal intercourse, but they can also be transferred through anal sex, oral sex, or skin-to-skin contact.

Men may believe that they would know if they had an STD. While most STDs do cause symptoms, many are easily mistaken for other conditions, and in some cases, there are no symptoms at all.

The penis is one area of the body that can provide clues as to whether a man has contracted an STD. Understanding the risks and knowing the signs and symptoms of common STDs in men is important if you are sexually active. Here are symptoms affecting the penis that could indicate an STD:

- **Discharge from the penis**—Men infected with gonorrhea may notice a thick white, yellow, or green discharge from the tip of their penis. Other symptoms can be pain with urination or in the urethra. Treatment for gonorrhea includes two drugs—a single dose of intramuscular ceftriaxone and oral azithromycin. These medications will stop the disease but not repair any permanent damage it caused.

- **Burning sensation when urinating**—Chlamydia often has few if any symptoms, but they usually include a burning sensation when urinating, a discharge from the penis, or pain and swelling in one or both testicles. If symptoms do appear, it may be several weeks after sex with an infected partner.

- **Sore on the penis**—Syphilis can appear on the penis as a hard, painless, dime-sized sore. There may also be swollen lymph nodes in the groin. Treatment is a single intramuscular injection of long-acting penicillin G benzathine.

- **Red bumps on the penis and scrotum**—Itchy, red bumps and nodules appearing in lines are signs of a scabies infection. Generally, scabies may not always be in a list of STDs, but because it can be spread through sexual contact, it can be classed as one. This common skin infestation may look like a rash, and if a man scratches the bumps, they can become infected with bacteria. Treatment requires a prescription cream or lotion.

- **Painful blisters or scabs on the penis**—Genital herpes can present as a cluster of painful or itchy red spots and small blisters on the penis. Men will notice itching or pain first, then blisters a day or two later. Unfortunately, there is no cure for herpes. Taking antiviral medications help shorten or prevent outbreaks. Also taking a daily antiviral medication can reduce transmission to a partner.

Best Practices for Preventing or Transmitting STDs

- **Abstinence**—The most reliable way to avoid infection is to not have sex.

- **Vaccination**—Safe and effective, the HPV vaccine can protect against some of the most common types of HPV.

- **Reducing number of sex partners**—You and your partner should get tested and share test results.

- **Mutual monogamy**—Agree to be sexually active with only one uninfected person.

- **Condom use**—Correctly and consistently using condoms is highly effective for reducing STD transmission.

Source: CDC.gov

SUMMARY

- Men should have a good understanding of both the external and internal male reproductive structures.

- The penis can be a good indicator of other health issues you may have and not know it.

- Erectile dysfunction is a quality-of-life issue. It often results from a significant health malady such as heart disease, hypertension, diabetes, osteoporosis, or vitamin D deficiency, as well as certain medications.

- A prolonged erection (lasting more than four hours) is called priapism and needs emergency medical intervention to prevent long-term consequences to a man's ability to achieve an erection.

- A curved, erect penis or a penis leaning to the right or left could indicate Peyronie's disease. Any changes in the penis like these need to be evaluated by a doctor.

- Premature ejaculation, while frustrating, is an easily treatable condition.

- Penile cancer, while rare, is best caught early to prevent permanent disfiguration or removal of part or all of the penis. Men should inspect their penis for any physical signs or symptoms of this disease.

- Men who are uncircumcised have a higher risk of balanitis, an infection of the glans of the penis. Practicing good hygiene by keeping the foreskin clean is one of the best ways to prevent this condition.

- Certain STDs directly affect the penis. Men need to take responsibility by protecting themselves and their partners from contracting or transmitting an STD.

CHAPTER 8

The Power of Sex on Men's Health

Approximately seventy-five years ago, a psychologist named Abraham Maslow came up with a list of basic human needs. These needs were not intended to be a recipe for happiness but were instead meant to describe people when they are in a long-term state of contentedness. This list, first published in the 1940s, is called the hierarchy of human needs and includes physiological needs (such as food, water, and sleep), safety, love and belonging, esteem, and self-actualization.[1]

This chapter will zero in on just one of these human needs, love/belonging—or to be blunt, sex and sexual intimacy. Few men would disagree that regular connection through physical touch and sex is important for not only maintaining a sense of well-being but also allowing for self-care. Every day, I see men who need their sexual issues addressed both physically and psychologically. My goal as a urologist is to steer men in the direction of gaining that sense of well-being and prioritizing self-care—and if sex is the motivator, that's even better.

What Is Men's Sexual Health?

Mr. Maslow was a smart and insightful man. He knew how important sex is to each of us. For men, sex probably registers a 12 on a scale of 1 to 10 in importance. From the time we wake up until we crawl into bed at night, sex frequently permeates our minds. There is surprisingly scant data on how often sexual thoughts pop into men's heads, but let's just agree, most of us think about it often.

Sex between humans is designed for two main reasons—the procreation of our species and pleasure. But a third reason really goes back to Maslow's hierarchy of human needs, and that is strengthening and cementing the bond between two people. Physical touch and intimacy between a man and his partner are powerful anecdotes for a range of physical, psychological, interpersonal, and social factors influencing his sexual health.

How do we define men's sexual health? In the clinical sense, optimal sexual health for men includes a healthy desire for sex or having a strong libido, and then the ability to get and sustain an erection for sexual intercourse. Having both a desire for sex and the ability to have sex largely depends on our mental and emotional health. If we are suffering mentally or emotionally—with stress, depression, and relationship issues, for example—we may also struggle sexually by experiencing low libido and/or erectile dysfunction.

Besides mental or emotional issues, physical factors also influence our sexual health. We may strongly desire sex, but physical factors that inhibit healthy sexual functioning may get in the way of good sex. These sex spoilers may include heart disease, diabetes, abnormally low testosterone, premature ejaculation, and urological surgeries.

Besides the Obvious, Why Is Sex So Good for Men?

Engaging in sexual activity is overwhelmingly pleasurable for men. The tremendous magnitude of complete bliss and euphoria makes us want to do it again and again.

What men may not know is the incredible favors sex is doing for our health. Keeping ourselves busy beneath the sheets has mental, emotional, and physical benefits that extend far beyond the bedroom. Thanks to this gift of nature, sex carries a lot of clout when it comes to our confidence, virility, and enjoyment of life.

So, just how beneficial is sexual activity for keeping yourself healthy? Here's a look at what it can do:

- **Reduces stress**—The act of intimacy is powerful stuff—touching, kissing, and holding one another not only feels good but also releases the hormones endorphins and oxytocin, which activate pleasure centers in the brain. This is why after a romp in bed, you feel more relaxed and at peace as you drift off to sleep. While stress and anxiety may not completely go away, you will feel better at least briefly, with an improved perspective on life.

- **Enhances immune system functioning**—Having sex at least once a week may help increase levels of immunoglobulin A (IgA), an antibody that plays a critical role in healthy immune functioning. When IgA levels are raised, our body is better able to fight off colds and flu by giving the immune system an extra boost.[2]

- **Improves physical fitness**—Ever wondered how much of a workout you get in between the sheets? Depending on how vigorous and energetic the sexual activity becomes, the average man may burn approximately 100 calories.[3] Not bad for a good time. Since the butt, back, and thighs get in on the action, some toning can be expected. Even the arms, legs, and abs can be sculpted by creative sexual positions.

- **Boosts sleep health**—A woman should not necessarily take offense if her man rolls over and falls fast asleep after lovemaking. We can blame it on two hormones—oxytocin (the love hormone), which increases, and cortisol (the stress hormone), which decreases. Basically, after reaching orgasm, we are feeling loved and less stressed, the perfect combo for inducing drowsiness and a very relaxed state of mind. This sleep-induced lull also leads to the all-important rapid eye movement (REM) sleep characterized by low muscle tone, quick eye movements, and dreams. Why is this important? REM sleep stimulates areas in your brain essential for learning and for making and retaining memories. This phase of sleep also allows the brain to exercise important neural connections key to mental and overall health and well-being.

- **Eases aches and pains**—Sex may not totally eliminate all aches and pains, but if you're feeling a little achy or headachy, sexual intimacy may be your fix. This is the prescription suggested from a study that showed sex did help some people experience less pain.[4] Why? Because reaching orgasm releases a flood of oxytocin and endorphins, helping ease annoying headaches and other pain, at least for a while.

- **Potentially lowers prostate cancer risk**—If you want to do whatever you can to avoid developing prostate cancer, start having frequent sex. Research has supported the notion that men who ejaculate at least twenty-one times a month are less likely to develop prostate cancer.[5] If you recall from chapter 6, one theory is that ejaculation may help clear the prostate of carcinogens or other harmful substances, but this is only based on an association. This advice does not advocate using sex as the only way to possibly prevent prostate cancer. But it could be fun to try—and if it's true, it's a welcome fringe benefit.

- **Improves heart health**—The number one killer of men in the United States is heart disease. Here's my prescription for avoiding it—eat a heart-healthy diet, exercise regularly, don't smoke, reduce stress, and have sex two to three times a week. That last suggestion you probably don't hear very often. Yet men who have sex two to three times a week have a lower rate of cardiovascular disease than men who have sex only a few times a month or less.[6] There are a couple of theories as to why frequent sex appears to improve heart health. One, sex is a type of physical activity, so it could give your heart a mini workout as your heart rate increases. Two, men engaging in frequent sex are likely to be in an intimate, loving relationship. Close bonds with a supportive partner makes for a healthy heart, both physically and emotionally, by easing stress levels.

- **Helps us look younger**—Want to turn back the clock? Then engage in coitus at least four times a week. The simple act and enjoyment of intimacy releases estrogen, testosterone, and the youthful-promoting hormone DHEA (dehy-droepiandrosterone), potentially making a man look seven to twelve years younger.[7]

- **Enhances self-esteem and intimacy**—Consistent sex involving mutual plea-sure promotes strong bonding between a couple. Thanks to a surge in oxytocin release at orgasm, feelings of affection, intimacy, and closeness are magnified. Just the act of sex improves your quality of life, helping you feel better about yourself, your partner, and life in general.

When Apprehension Overtakes Sexual Performance

There's a lot of social pressure on men to perform sexually. Most of us naturally think in terms of our "performance" in the bedroom—was it good or not? Did we help our partner reach climax? Did we last long enough, and did we perform up to par? Usually, these normal concerns aren't bothersome enough to prevent us from having sex. But some men are not so gung ho about hopping into bed. They approach sexual interludes with fear or uneasiness of what may or may not happen. This apprehension has a name—sexual performance anxiety.

Sexual performance anxiety is when a man feels enough tension or dread of sex to affect his ability to get aroused, even though he is physically healthy. The built-up anxiety can lead to erectile dysfunction, premature ejaculation, delayed or blocked ejaculation, and loss of libido. When a man is preoccupied with poor sexual performance, even when he is attracted to someone and wants to have sex, any negative sex-related thoughts may lead to this problem. Add to this scenario other pressures of life—worries about relationships, kids, work, and financial issues, which can potentially boil over into the bedroom—and he has created even more anxiety over his sexual abilities. Men of all ages and relationship sta-tuses can be affected when life gets stressful, so sexual performance anxiety may develop at any time.

Stress can have a strong grip on our general health and well-being, including our sex life. The body's main stress hormone—cortisol—is nature's built-in alarm system. It's best known for helping fuel your body's fight-or-flight instinct in a crisis. Your adrenal glands, which sit on top of your kidneys, are in charge of making cortisol. Most cells in your body have cortisol receptors, which receive and use the hormone in different ways. For instance, when your body is on high alert—maybe you've been involved in a car wreck or you're scrambling to get a work project done—cortisol can alter or shut down functions that get in the way of dealing with the stressful situation. On top of that, when cortisol is released, it floods the body and narrows the blood vessels. Guess what? Men need good blood flow to achieve an erection. Without it, sexual performance will fizzle.

If you're experiencing a less than satisfactory love life, you should first acknowledge the problem. Erectile dysfunction, premature ejaculation, and loss of libido can have many causes besides anxiety, but to know for sure, seek help from a doctor. If you haven't seen your doctor in more than a year, you should have a complete physical exam, including blood tests that check for any medical condition that could be the root cause.

If nothing medically or physically wrong is found, then it's time to focus on other possible reasons, including sexual performance anxiety. You may be referred to a therapist trained in treating sexual disorders. They can provide guidance on using various techniques to gain control of sexual-related anxiety.

Being open and honest with your partner is another way you can ease your worries over sexual performance. When you are forthcoming, it can actually bring you and your partner closer together and improve your sexual relationship. Sometimes finding other ways to be intimate without intercourse can help. We all know sexual intercourse is the home run of sexual intimacy, but sensual massages, taking a warm bath or shower together, or taking turns pleasuring each other with masturbation can take some of the pressure off performing sexually.

Sexually Transmitted Diseases—Recognizing and Protecting Yourself (and Others) from Them

Here's a reality to embrace—anyone having sex is at risk for contracting a sexually transmitted disease, or STD. Add to this fact that we already know men are notoriously bad about getting annual checkups and are unlikely to ask for STD testing. To make matters even worse, STDs in men are often "symptomless" or mistaken for other conditions. For these reasons alone, men should be especially observant of and educated in knowing the signs and symptoms of STDs. Let's take a look at common STDs.

Chlamydia

Every year, about 2.8 million Americans contract chlamydia. It is known as the "silent disease" because 50 percent of men and 75 percent of women will have no symptoms. Passed person to person during vaginal, anal, or oral sex, it can also be passed from mother to child during a vaginal delivery. The more sex partners a man has, the greater his risk of contracting it. In men, the infection can occur in the penis, throat, or anus, and if left untreated, it can result in serious reproductive and other health problems such as epididymitis, a painful condition of the testicles that can cause infertility.

Symptoms in men:

- Pain when urinating
- A green, white, or yellow discharge from the penis
- Swollen testicles

Hepatitis B

Hepatitis B is caused by a highly contagious virus that infects the liver, causing inflammation and damage. One method of transmission is through sexual activity, especially with multiple partners, by contact with blood or bodily fluids of someone infected. Symptoms are often mistaken for the flu, and if left untreated, the virus will continue to damage the liver. Hepatitis B will cause either an acute or a chronic infection. Acute hepatitis B is a short-term infection that doesn't require treatment for most healthy adults.[8] Chronic hepatitis B is a long-lasting infection in which the virus does not go away. The chronic form can lead to cirrhosis of the liver, liver failure, and liver cancer. You can protect yourself from hepatitis B by getting the hepatitis B vaccine, a series of three shots given over six months. To be fully protected, you must get all three shots.

Symptoms in men:

- Loss of appetite
- Feeling lethargic
- Low-grade fever
- Muscle and joint aches and pain
- Nausea or vomiting
- Jaundice (yellow hue to the skin and dark urine)

Gonorrhea

Transmitted through anal, oral, or vaginal sex, this bacterial STD affects the anus, throat, or urethra in men. Men who are not treated can have infertility complications, prostate inflammation, a scarred and narrowed urethra, and testicular or scrotal pain.

Symptoms in men:
- Burning sensation when urinating
- A white, yellow, or green discharge from the penis, usually appearing one to fourteen days after infection
- Painful or swollen testicles
- A red or swollen urethra
- A sore throat

Genital Herpes

One of the most common STDs in the United States is genital herpes, affecting more than one out of every six people ages fourteen to forty-nine.[9] Caused by the herpes simplex virus (HSV), this viral infection comes in two types—herpes simplex virus type 1 (HSV-1) and herpes simplex virus type 2 (HSV-2). HSV-1 causes oral herpes, which results in cold sores and fever blisters. Most genital herpes are caused by HSV-2, but both types can occur in either the genital or oral areas. The virus is transmitted through direct contact with the mouth or genitals of an infected person through sexual intercourse or oral sex and kissing.

Symptoms in men:
- Silent or no symptoms in up to two-thirds of cases
- Fever
- Headache
- Tiredness
- Body aches
- Swollen lymph nodes
- Sores, blisters, or ulcers inside or around the anus or around the buttocks and thighs
- Eye infection
- Eczema herpeticum

Human Papillomavirus (HPV)

Practically all sexually active people will get HPV unless they are vaccinated. Frequently passed through vaginal and anal sex, this virus lives in the skin or mucous membranes and can affect the genital areas of both men and women. There are about forty types of HPV, most of which go away on their own without causing any health problems.

Symptoms in men:

- Genital warts that may appear in or around the anus or on the penis, scrotum, groin, or thigh
- Precancerous changes in the anus or penis

To greatly reduce the incidence of STDs, you should be aware of these preventable diseases and practice protecting yourself and others from them. If more of us take precautionary steps, we can significantly reduce the number of people, including children and babies, who contract an STD.

The Seven Best Ways to Protect Yourself from an STD

- **Every time you have sex, practice safe sex.** Barrier methods such as condoms and dental dams may not be 100 percent STD proof but are better than nothing.
- **You and your partner should be tested regularly if in a new sexual relationship.** If you're already being treated for an STD, wait to resume sexual activity until treatment is done.
- **Have sex only in a monogamous relationship.**
- **Do not drink or use drugs before sex.** Clear thinking is required to make responsible choices. When you're under the influence, bad decisions such as having sex with someone you barely know could result in an STD.
- **Limit your sexual partners.** Each sexual partner increases your risk of being exposed to an STD. Be selective in choosing sexual partners, limiting yourself to those who share your sexual values.
- **Don't rely on the other person for protection.** You are responsible for your health. Sex should wait until both of you are protected.
- **Know the signs and symptoms of STDs.** The more you know, the better you can protect yourself.

Source: CDC.gov

When a Man's Sex Drive Suffers

Men hate to talk about it. Most find it embarrassing and distressing, to say the least. That's because in most relationships, men are typically viewed as the initiators of sex. So when they become more passive and disinterested in bedroom activities, partners take notice.

Loss of libido can happen to both men and women. It's not unusual for sex drives to vary during the course of our lives. But when sexual desire plummets out of nowhere, it begs the question, "Why?" And because men can be so tight-lipped about the situation, not only does their sex drive suffer, but their emotional health is likely taking a hit, too.

What does low libido look like? Does it extend beyond the bedroom? And is it a complete lack of sexual desire? There are warning signs associated with low libido; some men may exhibit many signs, while others may show just a couple. The important thing is to recognize the signs indicating that your normal sex life has noticeably changed.

Most of us know that sexual thoughts and desires begin outside the bedroom. It's the small yet powerful gestures such as kissing the neck, holding hands, or cuddling on the couch while watching TV that send subtle yet strong signals of, "I'm interested in becoming intimate with you." But if the only time you touch as a couple is in bed, this could be a clue of low sexual desire. Even if you do have sex, it may feel mechanical or routine, with little or no intimacy. This could be a sign of apathy toward sex or only a meager desire for it. If you've nosedived to having sex only once or twice a month—or less—that's a glaring clue something is wrong.

When your sex life has gone down the tubes, it's time to figure out why. Is your low sexual desire more of a physical, emotional, or medically related problem? The best way to investigate begins with a visit to your doctor. Discussing sexual problems can be uncomfortable, but all doctors have heard it before. To get your sex life back, make that appointment to discover the root cause.

Every man is different, and so are causes of low libido. For some men, it's erectile dysfunction or performance anxiety. By reviewing your physical and emotional health or making adjustments to your medications, your doctor can often resolve the problem. But if the problem stems from problems like stress in your marriage, money issues, child raising, or overwhelming anxiety or depression, these causes may take more time and energy to remedy.

Although lighting a spark to rekindle your libido may take time, it can be done. Frequency of sex is not the goal; instead, focus on quality to restore your feelings of anticipation, intimacy, and satisfaction. It helps to keep things real; in other words, not every sexual encounter has to be perfect. Learn to laugh, finding humor even in the bedroom. Part of the fun of sex is being able to be silly and fun loving with your partner, where all pressure is off and each of you is being satisfied.

Be sure to use your brain, too. An active imagination is a valuable gift for helping sparks fly in the bedroom and keeping the flames burning brightly. Fantasies are considered a good thing by most marriage therapists as long as both spouses agree to them.

Building anticipation throughout the day is a very useful tool for reviving sexual desire. While spontaneous sex is great, it's not always practical. Jobs, children, and household duties get in the way. What is practical is the buildup of anticipating sex later that night. Start off with a little longer than usual goodbye kiss in the morning, send a sexy text message partway through the day, come home with a bottle of wine, and play each other's favorite music at dinner. By the time you both jump into bed, sexual tension will be palpable.

Taking good care of your body physically pays off for a healthy sex life, too. Getting and staying in good shape benefits your body not only physically but also mentally and emotionally. Exercise is a must for relieving stress, burning extra calories, and building muscle. When you look and feel good, you have more vitality and confidence. This confidence in your appearance overflows into sexual confidence.

Having a social network of friends, not just a network of friends on social media, is also helpful. When both of you spend time together with friends for dinner or drinks, attending a sporting event, or going to the theater, you can see one another in a different social environment and admire how you each interact with other people. You'll then remember you why you fell in love with each other in the first place.

If you make any of these changes and your libido still doesn't return, it's time for professional help. Sex and marital specialists are trained for these issues and can be a lifesaver when the bedroom action is missing.

When a Man's Sex Drive *Doesn't* Suffer but Sex Is Painful

What? Sex can be painful for men? Yes, it can. This may surprise you since painful sex is associated more with women, usually due to vaginal dryness, thinning of the vaginal wall, endometriosis, pelvic inflammatory disease, and other conditions. While pain during sex is not as common in men, it can happen, turning your normally pleasurable encounter into unanticipated torment.

Pain during sexual intercourse is not normal for men and needs to be investigated by your doctor. Below are eight possible causes your doctor may explore and work with you to treat, some of which we've already discussed:

1. **Sexually transmitted diseases**, especially if not treated

2. **Peyronie's disease**, making sex difficult due to a curved penis

3. **Penis deformities** such as hypospadias, in which the urethra opening is on the underside of the penis

4. **Phimosis**, the inability to retract the skin covering the head of the penis, making the foreskin overly tight

5. **Priapism**, an erection lasting longer than four hours

6. **Allergies or sensitivities** to soaps, creams, or cologne applied to the genitals

7. **Urinary tract infections**, possibly leading to pain during ejaculation

8. **Prostatitis**, inflammation or infection of the prostate gland that results in painful erections

What Habits Make It Harder for Men to Conceive?

Here's what most of us expect about becoming parents—we get married and soon we're bringing home our first child, or at least we bring a baby home according to our planned timetable. However, life has a funny way of disrupting well-thought-out plans. Infertility—the inability to get pregnant after twelve months of regular, unprotected sexual intercourse—affects about one in eight American couples.[10] Having trouble conceiving can alter relationships and lead to anxiety, depression, and even blame.

The ability to create life is not a gift to take lightly. It's often taken for granted that conception will be easy when the time is right, and that if it doesn't happen as planned, it won't be the man's fault. Although "trouble" conceiving is usually blamed on a woman's infertility, men and women are equally responsible for an infertility diagnosis. According to the CDC's National Health Statistics Report, about one-third of cases are attributable to men, one-third are attributable to women, and the other one-third is a combination of both male and female factors or factors that cannot be identified.[11] Most cases of female infertility are caused by ovulation problems, while male infertility is usually related to low sperm count, poor sperm movement, or abnormal sperm shape.

Infertility in a man can sometimes result from certain unhealthy lifestyle habits that unknowingly harm his ability to reproduce. The healthier a man is, the healthier his sperm for conceiving a baby.

So what habits might reduce your chances of fathering a child? Here's a list of five not-so-healthy habits you can break to make conception easier:

1. **Smoking**—Plain and simple, don't smoke. Among countless other reasons, the nicotine and other harmful substances found in cigarettes have been linked to lowered sperm counts and may slow down sperm's ability to swim fast as they scramble to fertilize the egg.[12]

2. **Spending too much time on the laptop**—Technology may have overtaken our lives, but we don't want it to take over our sexual lives and our ability to procreate. Recently, there have been concerns about male infertility due to crotch overheating by laptops. Remember, there's a reason the testicles are outside the body—they need to be at least two degrees cooler than the rest of you. If they get overheated, especially regularly, this could affect fertility. Studies have found that laptop use (i.e., keeping a running laptop on your lap) can increase scrotal temperature by about five degrees Fahrenheit in one hour.[13] This heat, along with mixed evidence of electromagnetic frequencies (EMF) from devices like cell phones, may reduce sperm motility and damage DNA, but more research is needed to know anything conclusive.[14] Spending too much time in hot tubs, saunas, and other toasty places may also cause overheating that affects fertility.

3. **Avoiding foods high in lycopene**—Men who regularly consume foods rich in the phytochemical lycopene have higher sperm counts and faster sperm, sort of like Olympic swimmers.[15] This powerful antioxidant found in red fruits and vegetables such as watermelons, tomatoes, cherries, red peppers, and strawberries helps fight oxidative stress, which can contribute to poor sperm health.

4. **Gaining too much weight**—Even men need to reach a healthy body weight before women conceive. Emerging evidence is suggesting that obese men may experience increased infertility.[16] Carrying excess weight could impact male reproductive potential by reducing sperm quality and may lower the number of sperm or eliminate sperm production altogether.

5. **Smoking pot**—Regardless of the ever-widening acceptance of marijuana, there has been conflicting evidence on its effect on male fertility. One study concluded that men who regularly smoke pot or eat food containing cannabis

may have low sperm counts.[17] However, other studies have found just the opposite—that men who smoke pot may have higher concentrations and sperm counts than men who have never used pot.[18] Research suggests that the likely reason for this is actually related to testosterone and risk-taking: men with higher testosterone levels—who already tend to have higher semen quality and sperm counts—also tend to be risk takers and are therefore more likely to smoke marijuana. One thing is for sure—men should not start using pot to increase sperm count as the studies have only shown an association between these factors, not a causation.

Help! How Can I Boost Sexual Performance?

All men want to be thought of as a sexual dynamo in bed. For many men, enhancing sexual performance ranks mighty high on their priority list.

So, how should you evaluate your sexual performance when on the bedroom stage? What are the criteria of a great "performance"? Is it always based on your ability to get and keep an erection for intercourse? Do both you and your partner need to achieve orgasm simultaneously? Or is finding pure pleasure in sex based on how deep a mutually loving and physical relationship is? Depending on your health and situation in life, the answer can be "maybe" or "yes" to each question.

Most of us love sex so much we'd likely engage in this pleasurable experience just about every day of the week if we could, especially if everything were in tip-top condition and raring to go. However, if we neglect our health as the years roll by, we may discover the sex we enjoyed with abandon in our twenties is different from sex twenty years later.

Even if your sex life has fizzled a bit, don't despair. There's still time to take back this gift of life. On the other hand, if your bedroom activities are A-OK, now is the time to take steps to preserve and protect your sexual health before problems develop.

Boosting sexual performance while enhancing sexual health can both be achieved. It's simply a matter of making healthy habits a part of your life. Here are eight behaviors of sexually healthy men you can start working on now:

1. Exercise regularly and consistently.

Want to get it on? Then hit the gym, step out on the trail, jump in the pool, or hop on your bike. Living a sedentary lifestyle is a sex-life killer. Sitting around does nothing for maintaining muscle mass, keeping weight in check, increasing metabolism, or boosting energy. And if you think exercising is vain, rethink that notion. Think of it instead as long-term sex insurance that's there for you throughout the years. Men who work up a sweat doing cardiovascular training and strength training will be not only healthier but also sexier. Start moving more each day. At the very least, exercise releases endorphins, those feel-good hormones we talked about that help increase confidence, energy, and libido—everything men need for better and more frequent sex.

2. Feed your body wisely.

Take a look at your dinner plate. Does it look like what a registered dietitian would approve of, or does it resemble more of what you might buy at a football stadium, like burgers, brats, and chips? There's no truer statement than "you are what you eat." That's right, what's on your plate can affect your performance in bed. So fill your plate with foods brimming with nutrients, antioxidants, and fiber—they'll all keep your sexual engine running.

Every so often, men may need a little help increasing blood flow to the penis. Remember, without good blood flow, you can struggle to achieve and maintain an erection. Believe it or not, certain food choices may help:

- **Chilies and peppers**—Want things hot in the bedroom? Spice things up by eating chilies and peppers, which help blood flow by reducing hypertension and inflammation.
- **Onions and garlic**—Here's another pair known for improving blood circulation. Just don't forget to brush your teeth before showing your love.
- **Bananas**—A rich source of potassium, bananas can lower blood pressure, which improves blood flow while boosting sexual performance.
- **Eggs**—A naturally good source of protein and B vitamins, eggs also help balance hormone levels and therefore reduce stress, which improves your chance of getting an erection.

3. Exercise your love muscle.

Whoever figured out Kegel exercises for enhancing sexual fulfillment should have a statue erected of them. That's because performing Kegels are excellent for strengthening the pelvic floor's muscles, which connect the base of the penis with the tailbone (the same muscles that control urine flow through the urethra). The pelvic floor muscles act like a sling, holding up the internal organs and intestines.

Besides controlling urinary or fecal incontinence, Kegels can also be a main-stay treatment option for improved sexual functioning regarding both ED and premature ejaculation. Working the pelvic muscles not only strengthens those muscles but also supports erections by improving blood flow to the penis. One study found 40 percent of men ages twenty and older were able to kick ED completely by performing Kegels for six months. Another 35.5 percent significantly improved their symptoms.[19] What's more, your erections may look, well, more erect. In other words, instead of pointing down or straight forward, the penis is pointing up more toward the sky. Research has also shown for guys with premature ejaculation, Kegels can strengthen the urinary sphincter and other muscles that control ejaculation.[20] To properly do a Kegel, refer back to chapter 5.

4. Cut back on alcohol.

Here's a quick way to douse your sex life—start drinking heavily. The more you drink, the more at risk you are for ED, infertility, and changes in male secondary sex characteristics, such as less facial and chest hair.[21] While you may use or even depend on alcohol to feel sexier by lowering your inhibition, it also lowers your libido, making it harder to get an erection. Excessive alcohol use is also commonly involved in sexual assault or risky sexual activity, including unprotected

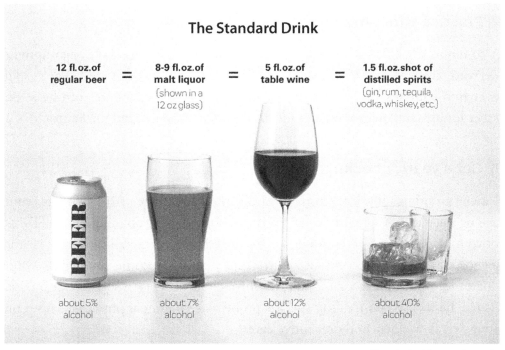

The Standard Drink

| 12 fl.oz. of regular beer | = | 8-9 fl.oz. of malt liquor (shown in a 12 oz glass) | = | 5 fl.oz. of table wine | = | 1.5 fl.oz. shot of distilled spirits (gin, rum, tequila, vodka, whiskey, etc.) |

about 5% alcohol   about 7% alcohol   about 12% alcohol   about 40% alcohol

Photo: Michael Shay @ Polara Studio

sex, sex with multiple partners, or sex with a partner at risk for sexually transmitted diseases.[22] If you choose to drink alcohol, always drink responsibly, and for men, that means consuming no more than two drinks a day (two 12-ounce beers, two 5-ounce glasses of wine, or two 1.5-ounce servings of spirits).

5. Stop smoking.

A significant cause of sexual dysfunction in men is smoking. Men who smoke are more likely to experience ED. Again, it goes back to good blood flow, which is necessary for achieving an erection. Years of dragging on a cigarette damages small arteries and therefore reduces blood flow, resulting in a penis that doesn't want to play.[23] As mentioned earlier, smoking can also reduce sperm count and quality.[24]

6. Stay away from illegal drugs.

While it's never a good idea to do illegal drugs, some men may believe it can enhance their sex life. They're wrong. Most illegal drugs have the opposite effects, often resulting in ED, lack of desire, and fatigue. Even prescribed medications can cause sexual issues, negatively affecting sexual arousal and performance. If this is the case, talk to your doctor about switching to a different medication.

7. Practice stress management.

A common sex killer is stress. Stress has a unique ability to make men uptight, nervous, anxious, and even exhausted. These stressful feelings are likely to spill over into your sex life. Practicing stress-management techniques can be a lifesaver for bringing relaxation and ultimately intimacy back into the bedroom.

8. Get a yearly checkup.

Having an annual physical exam is basic health maintenance 101. No matter your age or stage of life, a yearly checkup is essential to your ongoing health. Think of your primary care practitioner as your healthcare partner. That yearly visit is a good way for them to get to know you and vice versa. While you may see your doctor for minor illnesses and injuries throughout the year, those "sick care" visits will be focused on treating specific problems. An annual physical focuses on your overall wellness and preventive care.

Preventive care is one of the best ways to identify and treat health issues before they get worse. Annual physicals usually involve—depending on your age, lifestyle, and family history—screenings to check blood pressure, cholesterol, blood glucose, and body mass index. Your doctor will also review your vaccination history and may recommend getting vaccinated for the flu, pneumonia, HPV, shingles, and hepatitis B. Screenings for colon, lung, prostate, and skin cancer will be reviewed and recommended. It's simply the best way to catch anything you're unaware of and to discuss issues you're concerned about, such as your sex life or lack thereof.

Some Sex Advice for Men over Fifty

Do you see yourself as being "over the hill" after your fiftieth birthday? Do you consider it a halfway point in life, with fewer years ahead of you than behind you? It's easy to see why you might start feeling old when gray hair sprouts and wrinkles form, or when your muscles ache and your energy dwindles.

But worst of all are the problems involving sex. From low libido to erectile dysfunction, these sexual issues can throw a wrench into your sex life. How can you prevent them or turn things around?

First, you're not alone. I can tell you from the countless patients I've talked to that plenty of men around you share these feelings but often don't want to admit them. Some men may even consider this part of their life—their sexual side—to be a thing of the past. That's nonsense. Plenty of men who blew out fifty candles on their birthday cake years ago will tell you sex is not dead after you're fifty. In fact, many of them will say it's better than ever. If that's the case, what is their secret to a sensational sex life? What do they know that you need to know?

Here's a start—look down at your belly. What do you see…or not see? Does your belly hang over your belt so much that you can't see your feet? Carrying excess belly fat is no friend to your sex life. It influences your ability to achieve erections hard enough for intercourse. As we've discussed, excess weight often leads to atherosclerosis by reducing blood flow to the penis that's needed for an erection.

To assess whether your belly fat is at a healthy level, you need to know your waist circumference. To do this, wrap a cloth tape measure horizontally around the largest part of your belly—where your elbow bends at your waist. Keeping the tape snug but not to where it's compressing your skin, measure your waist after you breathe out. A waist circumference of forty inches or greater indicates too much of a type of fat called visceral fat, putting your health and sex life at risk. Visceral fat is stored in your abdominal cavity around many important organs, such as your liver, pancreas, and intestines. Often referred to as central obesity, visceral fat gives overweight and obese men a beer belly or an apple shape, which poses a greater risk for developing major chronic disease such as type 2 diabetes, heart disease, and stroke. Anyone who is obese is two to three times more likely to develop diabetes than someone of a normal weight. Remember, more than 50 percent of men with diabetes suffer from ED (chapter 7).

Aside from causing your libido to nosedive, plummeting testosterone levels can also make you less energetic. Men who used to work sunup to sundown would still have plenty of get-up-and-go in the bedroom, but nowadays, many men need an afternoon nap just to make it to dinnertime, so they forget about any hanky-panky later on.

Now that you know what may happen sexually once that fiftieth birthday comes and goes, what can you do to prevent anything from interrupting this intimate part of your life? Follow this advice:

- **Start with your physician.** If you want to put the spark back in your love life, have a frank discussion with your doctor about what's going on and how long you've had problems.

- **Have your heart functioning checked out.** If you have high blood pressure, high cholesterol, ED, or diabetes, get checked for heart disease.

- **Consider medication.** If ED is the issue, one of the first-line treatments for it is Viagra, Levitra, or Cialis. Each prescription can be very effective for helping you perform in bed and regain your sex life. A primary care physician or urologist can determine which medication is best for you.

- **Relax and make time for sex.** I've said it before—men who feel overwhelmed with numerous responsibilities and obligations often have little desire for sex. Prioritizing time to foster your sexual side with your partner can help you regain intimacy. By removing barriers that block you from nurturing a loving and meaningful relationship, you'll experience greater fulfillment and possibly the best sex of all.

SUMMARY

- Regular physical touch, including sex, is important for maintaining a sense of well-being and self-care.

- Optimal sexual health for men includes a healthy desire for sex and achieving an erection for sexual intercourse.

- Sexual activity has numerous benefits for men, including reduced stress, strengthened immunity, better sleep, and reduced risk of prostate cancer.

- Sexual performance anxiety can be overcome by addressing any associated medical or physical issues. Seeing a therapist who specializes in sexual disorders is another avenue you may need to consider.

- Recognizing signs and symptoms of STDs is important for protecting yourself and others.

- Loss of libido is not unusual in men. Recognizing why it may be happening is key to gaining control over it.

- One-third of infertility in couples is attributable to men, partly due to unhealthy habits.

- Sex can be painful even for men. Understanding the possible reasons why can be a first step toward fixing it.

- Sometimes a man's sex life can fizzle. To revive and boost sexual performance, you should follow some healthy behaviors, like exercising regularly and managing stress.

PART 3

Healthy Habits to Last a Lifetime

CHAPTER 9

Healthy Foods Make Healthy Men

There's no doubt that food and nutrition influences men's health. Before we start talking about nutrition, though, let me ask you this first: What is your definition of men's health? Are you full of energy and stamina, enjoying life to its fullest? Or do you feel lucky just to get through each day with minimal pain and few complaints?

As men, each of us has our own definition of health. As a physician, I would define men's health as being free of disease or disability along with a state of complete physical, mental, and social well-being. Of course, meeting these criteria 100 percent—especially 100 percent of the time—is rare. But it never hurts to strive to be our best—or at the very least, to make day-to-day choices promoting our health most of the time.

That's why thinking of the big picture, the overall lifetime of how we treat our body physically, emotionally, and mentally, adds up to what our own individual pictures of health will look like over time.

This section of the book looks at the big pillars that promote health and wellness over the course of your life. Forget about getting caught up in the latest new diet trend or fad. Walk away from quick fixes for anything from prostate health to sleep aids. What you need is smart, scientific, research-based evidence to help you regain and maintain good health. Focus on getting sufficient sleep, adding in more movement every day, reducing stress, refraining from illicit substances, and choosing an overall healthy eating pattern. Maybe these pillars are not considered sexy or attention grabbing, but trust me, they are considered the foundation of making you a healthy man for life. And trust me, healthy men are sexy men.

If I had to choose only one piece of advice for men to make tremendous strides in their health, it would be to eat highly nutritious foods. What you feed your body can be a make-or-break determining factor for either living a healthy, robust life or feeling sickly and lethargic. Obviously, many factors contribute to our overall well-being, but food choices rank high in promoting good health.

For something that is a basic human need, what we buy at the grocery store to feed our body is not necessarily instinctual. If motivation always moved us to choose healthy, nourishing foods, we'd be set. But with more than thirty thousand food items sold in the average grocery store, each one vying for your attention, it's a dicey proposition.[1] Bargains on chips, soda, and hot dogs may be all it takes to make unhealthy choices. To start incorporating healthier choices into your diet, you first need to get a better idea of what healthy foods are and what eating well looks like.

A Lifetime of Nutrient Nourishment

Throughout your lifetime, your food choices will have a monumental overall impact on your health. Each day, you make numerous decisions on what to eat. Depending on the nutrient composition of the food, its nutritional value will likely have cumulative effects on your body. Basically, whatever foods you eat daily will determine the nutrients you are feeding your body. But what exactly are nutrients, anyway?

Nutrients are components found within food that are necessary for your body to function properly. Nutrients provide us with energy, fueling our body to stay alert all day at work or to work out at the gym. Nutrients not only help us grow from infancy to adulthood, but they are also integral in maintaining and repairing body tissue, which is necessary for healing wounds. When you're lacking sufficient nutrients, you'll notice the effects—feeling sluggish or having a weakened immune system, for example.

The human body requires six different kinds of nutrients: carbohydrates, protein, fat, vitamins, minerals, and water. The first three—carbohydrates, protein, and fat—are also known as the energy-yielding or calorie-yielding nutrients, meaning they supply your body energy, or calories (in the world of nutrition, these terms are synonymous). These three nutrients are also called *macronutrients* (*macro* meaning "large") because they are necessary in large amounts for the human body. Every single bite of food we eat, whether it's a grilled cheese sandwich or a green salad, contains a proportion or combination of different macronutrients. Much of your foods are composed of all three macronutrients. A hamburger on a bun, for example, would be a combination of carbohydrates in the bun along with protein and fat in the meat. Some foods such as oils (e.g., olive or canola) are composed of 100 percent fat, whereas a spoonful of granulated sugar is 100 percent carbohydrate. Each of the macronutrients not only supplies energy but also has various other functions in the body, from providing materials that form structures of body tissue to helping absorb other nutrients from our food.

Vitamins and minerals are referred to as *micronutrients* (*micro* meaning "small") as they are needed by your body in only trace amounts—in other words, the body doesn't require much of them to do its work.

Micronutrients do not provide the body with energy or calories. Their main function is to act as regulators. As regulators, vitamins and minerals assist and are heavily involved in every process necessary to maintain life: digesting food, moving muscles, disposing wastes, growing new tissues, healing wounds, and extracting energy from carbohydrates, fat, and protein.

The sixth nutrient—water—also does not provide calories but is crucial for us just to remain alive. Water has numerous functions in our body, such as acting as a lubricant, cleansing the blood of waste, transporting nutrients, and regulating body temperature. Most of us could survive several weeks without food but no more than a few days without water. Your body does not make or store water. Whatever water you lose daily from sweating, urinating, or breathing must be replaced by either drinking it or by consuming other fluids and food sources containing it.

Ideally, most of us should eat foods high in nutrient density. Nutrient density is a measure of nutrients provided per calorie of food. In other words, a nutrient-dense food provides vitamins, minerals, and other beneficial substances with relatively few calories. For example, if you wanted to increase your calcium intake, a couple of food choices supplying this mineral would be ice cream and 1 percent low-fat milk. Do you choose a cup of premium ice cream containing more than 350 calories or a cup of 1 percent milk with only 100 calories and almost double the calcium? It's clear which one is more nutrient dense.

What about Calories? How Many Do I Need?

Men are notorious for focusing on calories, whether for weight loss or weight maintenance. The total number of calories you require each day depends on certain factors, such as your age, height, current weight, and level of physical activity. Other factors affecting your calorie needs may be influenced by certain disease conditions or malnutrition.

For adult men, the range of calories you consume should be around 2,000 to 3,000 per day. The low end is recommended for sedentary men, while the high end is for more active men. As men (and women) age, we reduce the rate at which we burn calories, so our calorie needs generally decrease. For men who want to maintain weight, the following guidelines provide calorie estimates based on age and physical activity levels:

Calorie Needs for Men Based on Age and Activity Level			
Age	Sedentary	Moderately Active	Active
19–20	2,600	2,800	3,000
21–25	2,400	2,800	3,000
26–35	2,400	2,600	3,000
36–40	2,400	2,600	2,800
41–45	2,200	2,600	2,800
46–55	2,200	2,400	2,800
56–60	2,200	2,400	2,600
61–65	2,000	2,400	2,600
66–75	2,000	2,200	2,600
76 and up	2,000	2,200	2,400

Source: 2015–2020 Dietary Guidelines for Americans

Notes: Sedentary activity includes only the physical activity of independent living; *moderately active* includes physical activity equal to walking about 1.5 to 3 miles a day at 3–4 miles per hour (mph), plus activities of independent living; and *active* includes physical activity equal to walking more than 3 miles per day at 3–4 mph, plus activities of independent living.

Simplifying Healthy Food Choices through Macronutrients

Now that you're familiar with macronutrients and micronutrients and have a better idea of your calorie needs, let's focus on choosing the best foods to fuel your body. The best way to make smart selections is to categorize foods into the three macronutrients—carbohydrates, protein, and fat.

Carbohydrates

The key to choosing healthy carbohydrates is to think fiber. Few Americans consume enough fiber. The Dietary Reference Intakes (DRI) recommends 38 grams a day for men—more than twice the average intake of only 15 grams. Do not skimp on fiber. Fiber, the indigestible parts of plant foods—think of the thin strands in celery or the edible peels of fruit—plays a vital role in protecting you from heart disease, cancer, and digestive problems. Depending on the type—soluble or insoluble—it lowers cholesterol, helps with weight control, and regulates blood sugar.

Men's Daily Carbohydrate Needs

The Dietary Guidelines for Americans from the U.S. Department of Health and Human Services recommends 45 to 65 percent of total daily calories from carbohydrates. For a man following a 2,000-calorie diet, this means between 900 and 1,300 calories should come from carbohydrates, or 225 to 325 grams daily since carbohydrates contain 4 calories per gram. Some men may need fewer carbohydrates depending on medical circumstances.

Found only in plant-based foods (fruits, vegetables, beans, seeds, nuts, whole grains), fiber is an element our body does not digest. Instead, fiber passes quickly through your digestive tract, mostly intact, which is a good thing. Undigested fiber creates bulk, which physically helps move stools and harmful carcinogens through your digestive tract and out your body. Consuming a high-fiber diet has been shown to reduce the risk of various health conditions, including heart disease, diabetes, diverticular disease, constipation, and colon cancer.[2] Our digestive system relies on fiber for sweeping up and out particles and compounds that could potentially cause health issues in the small and large intestine.

Speaking of the health of our digestive tract, did you know this part of our body is home to about one hundred trillion bacteria made up of thousands of different species? This living, breathing, highly complex ecosystem that lives in harmony with us weighs on average about 4.5 pounds. Also known as the gut microbiome or gut flora, this ecosystem is now recognized as an additional organ system important in digestive health—it aids in metabolizing and absorbing nutrients from food, produces vitamin K, and acts as a protective barrier against intestinal infections, among other roles. These dynamic organisms vary by strain from one person to the next so that each one of us has our own unique microbiota. More and more studies are finding this community of gut microbiota may play a role in enhancing our immune functioning while reducing our risk of cancer, heart disease, rheumatoid arthritis, and other health conditions.[3]

Time for a Gut Check

A healthy gut microbiome doesn't just happen—it needs to be well fed to keep the good bacteria plentiful. When your gut is happy, you are happy. Here's how you can help make that happen:

1. Do not overuse antibiotics as that can deplete good gut bacteria.

2. Eat more fermented foods. Bacteria are living organisms that need to eat, and fermented foods encourage a diverse ecosystem. Naturally fermented foods include sauerkraut, pickles, miso, Greek yogurt, and kefir.

3. Eat a high-fiber diet:

   • Add beans or lentils to soups and salads

   • Add fruit to oatmeal and yogurt

   • Twenty-four almonds have 4 g fiber

   • 1 cup peas have 9 g fiber

   • 1 cup barley has 6 g fiber

Fiber plays a special role in boosting your gut flora. The good bugs in your microbiota thrive on certain types of fiber found in fruits, vegetables, nuts, seeds, and whole grains. For example, inulin is a fiber found in high concentrations in onions, asparagus, and garlic. As fiber passes undigested through the small intestine into the colon, the bacteria there start to ferment it. As the organisms munch away, the fiber is converted into chemicals. This process helps lower inflammation while sealing the gut lining—which is necessary to protect bacteria from leaching from the intestines into the bloodstream, possibly leading to bloating, gas, or cramps, for example.

Here's another reason eating more fiber is good for gut health—studies have shown switching to either a plant-based or an animal-based diet can significantly affect the number and type of bacteria. After just four days of increasing fiber from plant-based foods, the activity of fiber-fermenting bacteria increases, lowering your gut's pH and balancing your good bacteria. So, if you like meat, be mindful of the portion size, and be sure to eat a dark leafy green salad filled with vegetables along with it.[4]

Fiber in food is often categorized as either soluble or insoluble. Soluble fiber does just what it sounds like—it easily dissolves in water into a gel-like consistency.

Best known for its ability to lower blood glucose and blood cholesterol levels, improve weight management, and promote colon health, soluble fiber is found in oats, barley, legumes, okra, apples, and citrus fruits. Insoluble fiber does not dissolve in water or form a gel, and it is poorly fermented. If you're looking to prevent constipation and hemorrhoids and lower your risk of colon and rectal cancers, insoluble fiber is your answer. Find it in brown rice, seeds, fruits, and vegetables such as cabbage, carrots, Brussels sprouts, and whole grains. Most foods that contain fiber have a combination of both soluble and insoluble fibers.

Besides being the body's main energy source (your brain requires a steady supply of glucose, a type of sugar from carbohydrates), fiber-rich carbohydrate foods are your go-to for maintaining a healthy body weight. Let's take a look at high-fiber foods to choose from each day:

High-Fiber Foods		
Fruit	**Serving Size**	**Total Fiber (Grams)**
Raspberries	1 cup	8
Pear	1 medium	6
Apple, with skin	1 medium	4.5
Banana	1 medium	3
Orange	1 medium	3
Strawberries	1 cup	3
Vegetables	**Serving Size**	**Total Fiber (Grams)**
Green peas, cooked	1 cup	9
Broccoli	1 cup	5
Turnip greens, boiled	1 cup	5
Brussels sprouts	1 cup	4
Potato, with skin, baked	1 medium	4
Sweet corn, boiled	1 cup	3.5
Cauliflower, raw	1 cup, chopped	2
Carrot, raw	1 medium	1.5

Continued on next page

Grains	Serving Size	Total Fiber (Grams)
Whole wheat spaghetti, cooked	1 cup	6
Barley, pearled, cooked	1 cup	6
Bran flakes	3/4 cup	5.5
Quinoa, cooked	1 cup	5
Oat bran muffin	1 medium	5
Oatmeal, old-fashioned	1 cup	5
Popcorn, air popped	3 cups	3.5
Brown rice, cooked	1 cup	3.5
Whole wheat bread	1 slice	2

Legumes, Nuts, and Seeds	Serving Size	Total Fiber (Grams)
Split peas, cooked	1 cup	16
Lentils, cooked	1 cup	15.5
Chia seeds	1 ounce or 2 tablespoons	10
Edamame	1/2 cup	6
Black beans, canned	1/2 cup	5
Kidney beans, canned	1/2 cup	5
Almonds	1/2 cup	4
Chickpeas, canned	1/2 cup	4
Pistachios, without shells	1/4 cup	3
Sunflower seed kernels	1/4 cup	3
Brazil nuts	Six nuts	2
Pumpkin seeds	1/4 cup	2
Walnuts	1/4 cup	2

Source: Nutritiondata.self.com

Protein

Women may crave carbs, but men are infatuated with protein. We obsess over the amount, the quality, and where our proteins come from, and we faithfully follow diets based on colossal amounts of this nutrient. Why? We see protein as our ticket to a lean yet muscle-bound body boosting strength and vitality. But is protein the answer to improving our bodily concerns?

Protein is an amazing and versatile nutrient. Named after the Greek word *proteos* (meaning of "prime importance"), protein is composed of building blocks called amino acids. There are twenty different amino acids—eleven of which our body makes on its own, and nine of which are not made by our body (called essential amino acids) and therefore have to be obtained from our food. Protein deserves its nomenclature due to its vast role in making us who we are and how we function. From healing wounds to making enzymes, antibodies, and hormones, to transporting lipids, vitamins, minerals, and oxygen, to maintaining our fluid and electrolyte balance, to clotting the blood from an injury so we don't bleed to death, protein is a busy nutrient. And one more thing—protein is an integral component of our teeth, bones, skin, tendons, muscles, cartilage, blood vessels, and other tissues. All are important structures to the workings of a healthy body.

Are huge amounts of protein a good idea?

While most men rank protein as their top nutrient concern, few of us are deficient in it. We often consume large amounts of protein, especially those of us who are into fitness. After all, it makes us feel full, which helps with weight loss, and it works to build and maintain muscle mass. It's true that muscle contains about 40 percent of the protein in the human body. This has led people to believe that eating extra protein correlates directly to building large muscles. Sorry, guys, but wolfing down extra protein by itself does not magically build bulging muscles. What will enhance your prospects of gaining muscle mass is to eat adequate amounts of protein while focusing on regular weekly sessions of resistance training. Those food sources of protein are crucial in the recovery phase of working out and rebuilding muscle afterward.

The Recommended Dietary Allowance (RDA) for protein each day is 10 to 35 percent of total calories for adults.[5] Research shows no benefit to eating more protein than this amount.[6] In fact, eating a high-protein diet can lead to an unbalanced diet. Filling your plate with protein all day every day often replaces other high-quality foods your body needs to function properly. These foods include disease-fighting fruits and vegetables, heart-healthy fats, and whole grains that aid in digestion and weight loss. Anytime you overemphasize one macronutrient at the expense of the others, it can lead to deficiencies in vital nutrients. For example, if 60 percent of your diet is composed of protein with only 20 percent fat and 20 percent carbohydrates, you'll be denying your body of B vitamins, fiber, and extra energy that you would normally get in a moderate-carbohydrate diet.

Protein Recommendations for Men

- Protein should be 10 to 35 percent of total calories per the Dietary Reference Intakes (DRI) recommendation.

- The DRI recommendation is 0.8 g/protein per kilogram of body weight, or 0.37 g/protein per pound of body weight. Divide weight in pounds by 2.2 to convert to kilograms, or multiply weight in kilograms by 2.2 to convert to pounds. For example, if you weigh 70 kg (154 lb.), the DRI is approximately 57 g/protein per day.

- Older adults may need 1.0–1.2 g/protein per kilogram of body weight to preserve muscle mass.

- Endurance athletes may benefit from 1.2–1.4 g per kilogram of body weight.

- Strength athletes may benefit from 1.2–1.7 g per kilogram of body weight.

Source: The Academy of Nutrition and Dietetics, Dietitians of Canada, and the American College of Sports Medicine

Another way to look at protein intake is to take the focus off the *amount* and instead focus on *when* you eat it. The human body does not store protein like it does carbohydrates and fat. So once the body's needs are met, any extra protein is used for energy or stored as fat. Excess carbohydrates are stored in either muscles or the liver as glycogen, and once those are full, the rest is stored in adipose (fat) tissue. Extra fat your body can't use at a particular time also gets packed away in adipose tissue. This means your body has no storage space for extra protein when you need it for various functions—and it's also why research shows it's a bad idea to slam down a huge amount of protein in one sitting to try to build muscle. The best way to make sure you have sufficient protein available throughout each day is to spread your intake of this nutrient over your meals and snacks.

Remember how protein is composed of amino acids, building blocks for various needs like muscle building? Research has shown that aiming for about 25 to 30 grams of protein per meal and about 10 to 15 grams of protein per snack results in having those amino acids available throughout the day whenever your body needs them. Rather than skimping on protein at breakfast or lunch (when we normally eat an average of 10 and 20 grams, respectively) and eating most of it at dinner (when we typically eat 60-plus grams), spread out your intake to maximize the use of amino acids for building muscle. This same research also found that people who ate 12 ounces of beef (about 85 grams of protein) did not experience any greater benefits in muscle building than those who ate 4 ounces of beef (29 grams of protein), or roughly a palm-sized portion.[7] The extra protein from a 12-ounce steak (that is, anything more than 30 grams) will only get socked away in your adipose tissue and not your muscles.

Older adults may also benefit from proportionally more protein in their diets—evenly distributed over the day—for muscle health. Aging means loss of muscle mass known as sarcopenia. After about age fifty, we lose 0.5 percent to 2 percent of total muscle mass each year. This age-related muscle-mass loss can begin at even younger ages if low protein intake is paired with inactivity. This is why eating a meal with 4 to 5 ounces of high-quality protein—a palm-sized portion—will fill up your protein tank.

Add high-quality protein to your meal

High-quality protein comes from animal sources—beef, poultry, fish, pork, lamb, eggs, milk, and cheese. Animal foods contain all nine essential amino acids in the right proportion your body needs—they are composed of blood, bone, and tissue just like us. However, there is one exception of a plant-based source of protein that also contains all nine amino acids—soybeans.

For vegans, consuming a plant-based diet is very healthy and can still allow you to get the recommended protein intake. Good plant-based sources of protein include soy products, lentils, beans, grains, nuts, and seeds. It is important to know, however, that protein found in plant-based foods is encased in plant cell walls, making it difficult for our body to penetrate and digest it. Although plant-based proteins do not contain all nine essential amino acids, as long as vegans include a variety of plant-based sources of protein throughout the day, they can meet their protein needs adequately without developing a deficiency.

High-Protein Foods		
Food	Serving Size	Total Protein (Grams)
Egg	1 large whole	7
Cottage cheese	1/2 cup	12
Greek yogurt	1/2–1 cup	15–20
Cheese	1 ounce	6–10
Milk	1 cup	8

Continued on next page

Food	Serving Size	Total Protein (Grams)
Tuna, salmon, haddock, or trout	4 ounces	22–27
Turkey or chicken	4-ounce breast	25
Red meat—beef, pork, or lamb	4 ounces	25–30
Nuts—depending on type	1 ounce	2–6
Beans, cooked	1/2 cup	10
Lentils, cooked	1/2 cup	12
Split peas, cooked	1/2 cup	12
Tofu	1/2 cup	10
Edamame	1/2 cup	11

Source: Nutritiondata.self.com

Fat

Here's a fact most of us agree on—fat in our food makes eating pleasurable. From the smooth texture and rich taste of fat in ice cream to the unique flavor of olive oil in salads and the smell of bacon sizzling in a pan, fat is special. Life without it just wouldn't be the same.

But wait a minute—aren't we supposed to get rid of fat in our diet? Isn't fat bad for us? Not necessarily. In fact, fats are a valuable and necessary nutrient for us, but it all boils down to quality and quantity.

Fats, just like carbohydrates and protein, provide calories we need for energy, but they contain more than twice the amount of those two macronutrients: fats provide nine calories per gram, while carbohydrates and protein each provide four calories per gram. That's why following a high-fat diet can result in weight gain.

However, fat also helps keep us healthy. It's our major form of stored energy and a major material of cell membranes. We need fat to absorb vitamins; maintain healthy skin; insulate the body; act as a protective cushion for our bones, organs, and nerves; help us feel fuller longer; and make estrogen and testosterone. Even the human brain is composed of 60 percent fat.

How do I choose healthy fats?

For years, we were told to reduce fat in our diet. Now, things have flip-flopped, and we're told not all fat is bad. In fact, quality, healthy fats support good health without harming it. In other words, eating nutritiously does not mean cutting out all fats. Rather, your goal is to try to get 20 to 35 percent of your total daily calories from healthy fats and fewer than 10 percent of calories per day from unhealthy fats. Let's look at those good fats and not-so-healthy fats:

Unhealthy fats: saturated and trans fats—Saturated fats are typically solid at room temperature. They mainly come from animal products such as pork, beef, poultry, and dairy along with many snack products. High saturated fat intake is linked with higher levels of LDL (bad) cholesterol, which clogs arteries and leads to heart disease.

Trans fats are created when food manufacturers change a liquid fat (oil) into a solid fat. This process is called hydrogenation, so when an ingredient listed on a Nutrition Facts label states "hydrogenated" or "partially hydrogenated," those contain trans fat. Trans fats are considered even worse than saturated fat—they increase the risk of heart disease by lowering HDL (good) cholesterol while raising LDL cholesterol. The good news is that in 2015, the Food and Drug Administration ruled trans fats unsafe to eat.[8] Once ubiquitous in everything from frozen pizza to coffee creamer to microwave popcorn, artificial trans fats are thankfully being phased out of the American food supply.

Foods Rich in Saturated and Trans Fats	
Saturated Fats (Aim for < 10 Percent of Total Calories)	Trans Fats (Aim for 0 Percent of Total Calories)
• Whole milk	• Margarine
• Cream	• Cookies and cakes
• Ice cream	• French fries
• Whole-milk cheeses	• Fried onion rings
• Meats like beef, poultry with skin, pork, and lamb	• Donuts
• Sausage, bacon, hot dogs, and other processed meats	
• Butter and stick margarine	
• Tropical oils like coconut and palm kernel oil	
• Cakes, cookies, and some snack foods	
• Pizza, casseroles, burgers, tacos, and some sandwiches	

Source: Nutrition Concepts and Controversies

Healthy fats: monounsaturated and polyunsaturated fats/omega-3 fats— Monounsaturated fats are a type of fat found to help lower the risk of heart disease by lowering total cholesterol and LDL cholesterol while maintaining or improving HDL cholesterol. They may also improve the function of blood vessels and may benefit insulin levels and blood sugar control.

Polyunsaturated fats are another type of healthy fat mostly found in vegetable oils, walnuts, and fish. Omega-3 fats are a type of polyunsaturated fat offering health benefits such as helping your brain and nervous system to function normally, lowering cholesterol to support heart health, protecting against dry eye disease, and reducing inflammation in the body. There are three different types of omega-3 fats:

- ALA, or alpha-linolenic acid—found in plant oils such as canola oil, nuts such as walnuts, seeds such as flaxseed, and soy foods
- DHA, or docosahexaenoic acid—found mainly in fish and other seafood
- EPA, or eicosapentaenoic acid—found mainly in fish and other seafood

Your body can't make omega-3 fats, so you must get them from food. There are both natural food sources and certain foods fortified with omega-3 fats, like eggs, milk, and soy drinks. Your body can convert ALA you get from food into DHA and EPA but only in limited amounts. If you don't eat many foods containing omega-3s and think you would benefit from a supplement, talk to your healthcare provider first.

Foods Rich in Monounsaturated, Polyunsaturated, and Omega-3 Fats		
Monounsaturated Fats	**Polyunsaturated Fats**	**Omega-3 Fats**
• Nuts such as almonds, cashews, pecans, pistachios, and macadamias • Olive, canola, and peanut oils • Avocados • Nut butters like peanut or almond • Olives	• Walnuts • Sunflower and flaxseeds • Corn, soybean, sunflower, and safflower oils	• Salmon • Herring • Sardines • Lake trout • Atlantic or Pacific mackerel • Walnuts • Flaxseeds • Chia seeds • Hemp seeds • Eggs—if hens are fed a diet high in omega-3s

Source: Nutrition Concepts and Controversies

Easy ideas for including more healthy fats in your diet

Getting enough healthy fats into your diet doesn't have to be complicated, unappetizing, or time consuming. Here are a few simple ways to work them in daily:

- Combine nuts, seeds, dry cereal, and dried fruit for a snack mix.
- Use soft margarine as a substitute for butter. Look for 0 grams trans fat on the Nutrition Facts label.
- Enjoy a handful of nuts instead of chips or other fried snacks.
- Add chia, hemp, or flaxseeds to Greek yogurt, baked goods, or whole grain breakfast cereal.
- Add nuts to a salad and use an olive oil and vinegar dressing.
- Have a fruit salad instead of ice cream for dessert.
- Add avocado to a smoothie or salad, or use it in place of butter on toast.

Ten Health-Maximizing Foods for Men

Now that you have a clearer picture of what eating a nutritious diet looks like, I want to bring up an important topic: superfoods. Whether you want to call these ten foods superfoods is up to you. What I will say is there are certain foods that stand out in what they can offer healthwise. While there are dozens of other foods not on this list that can also boost your health, these ten pack the biggest punch.

1. **Fatty fish**—If heart health matters to you, your catch of the day should include salmon, tuna, halibut, lake trout, and sardines, all rich in omega-3s. Looking to lower your triglyceride level and blood pressure, or reduce blood clotting and your risk of a stroke? Make sure to have two or three 3-ounce servings each week of broiled or baked fish.

2. **Berries and tart cherries**—Some type of berry should always be in your kitchen. Blueberries, strawberries, raspberries, blackberries, and other berries are loaded with antioxidants, possibly helping to lower cancer risk while improving memory and concentration. Tart cherries are rich in anthocyanins and bioflavonoids, which may relieve pain from arthritis, gout, and even sore muscles. These same compounds may reduce migraine headaches and eliminate byproducts of oxidative stress to slow the aging process. Trouble sleeping? Choose cherries. They naturally contain melatonin, which improves your body's circadian rhythm.

3. **Tomato sauce**—Tomatoes are rich in the phytochemical lycopene, which becomes more available in your body when tomatoes are cooked or processed into tomato sauce or tomato paste.

4. **Lean red meat**—Packed with protein, iron, zinc, and vitamin B12, lean red meat also contains an amino acid called leucine, a key muscle-building component. The key to choosing healthy cuts of red meat is to look for the words *loin* or *round* on the package (e.g., *eye of round* or *top sirloin*). A 3-to-4-ounce serving size (the size of the palm of your hand) twice a week is sufficient.

5. **Dark chocolate**—Really, chocolate? Yes, but only dark chocolate with a cacao content of at least 70 percent or higher. A high cacao content provides flavonoids, an antioxidant-rich plant nutrient. Flavanols, the main type of flavonoids found in cocoa and chocolate, may influence vascular health by lowering blood pressure, improving blood flow to the brain and heart, and making blood platelets less sticky and able to clot. Enjoy moderate portions of dark chocolate, like a 1-ounce square, a few times per week.

6. **Orange and leafy green vegetables**—Talk about health foods! The eye-popping colors of sweet potatoes, carrots, peppers, spinach, kale, and collard greens, to name a few, should be in your grocery cart every week. Orange vegetables are excellent sources of beta-carotene, lutein, and vitamin C, all of which may reduce your risk of prostate cancer. Leafy greens also protect the prostate and are loaded with lutein and zeaxanthin, nutrients necessary to prevent cataracts and age-related macular degeneration.

7. **Prunes, figs, and dates**—Do not overlook this trio. Prunes are often a go-to laxative and are considered even more effective than psyllium in this regard. That's because they contain sorbitol, a natural sugar that pulls moisture into the digestive tract, softening stools and reducing constipation. And prunes are rich in manganese—which protects us from free radical damage—and in iron, a mineral necessary for carrying oxygen and enhancing our immune systems. One of the oldest-known fruits, figs are loaded with fiber—four figs provide 5 grams. Those same four figs also provide a healthy dose of potassium—240 mg—which helps lower blood pressure and therefore protects against stroke and heart disease. Dates are also rich in potassium and fiber. Plus, dates contain magnesium, a mineral essential for bone growth, and the mineral copper, required for producing red blood cells.

8. **Milk and Greek yogurt**—The dairy aisle is your stop for muscle-building food. Like red meat, both milk and Greek yogurt contain leucine, which helps make them excellent sources of protein—8 grams in one cup of milk and anywhere from 10 to 20 grams in a cup of yogurt. Greek yogurt also contains live bacteria, helping feed your gut microbiome to keep your digestive system running smoothly.

9. **Ancient grains**—Tired of rice or whole wheat pastas? It's time to discover ancient grains. Amaranth, teff, farro, freekeh, buckwheat, and wheat berries are just a few heritage grains, or ancient grains, providing excellent sources of not only energy but also protein, fiber, calcium, magnesium, iron, potassium, and zinc. What makes these grains especially nutritious is they are often in their whole form with all three parts of a grain kernel—bran, germ, and endosperm—intact.

10. **Almonds, walnuts, and pistachios**—A daily dose of nuts may determine what diseases you may or may not develop. A study from the Harvard School of Public Health showed those who ate a handful each day reduced their risk of both cardiovascular disease and cancer.[9] Need a food to fuel high-energy demands of physical activity? Nuts are the answer, along with helping reduce obesity and high blood pressure. Most are high in heart-healthy fat, vitamin E, magnesium, selenium, fiber, and protein, offering benefits such as improving cholesterol, metabolism, and eye health. Also choose from cashews, Brazil nuts, hazelnuts, and peanuts.

Five Foods That Harm Men's Health

Okay, so you're that guy who works out at least three times a week, doesn't smoke, and for the most part, keeps calm when life gets complicated. Basically, you're leading a fairly healthy lifestyle that should reward you with being able to avoid most chronic diseases.

But there's one thing you've been neglecting—eating healthy. Instead of eating foods that fuel your body with vital nutrients like antioxidants, vitamins and minerals, and fiber, you've been eating one too many cheeseburgers and fries… and it's beginning to show.

Here's a look at five types of food men tend to indulge in but should rarely eat instead:

1. **Junk food/highly processed foods**—A steady diet of chips, burgers, sausages, donuts, cookies, and all other overly sugared, high-sodium, high-fat foods is not good for anyone—no matter your age, gender, or level of activity. These highly processed concoctions can change the course of your life by raising your risk of heart disease, certain types of cancer, high blood pressure, obesity, and diabetes. Maybe when you were young you could get by with this type of unhealthy eating. But now, too many brats, unhealthy oils, and sodium-packed foods can take their toll. Foods like this can result in rapid weight gain, poor digestion, sluggishness, and lack of energy.

2. **Canned soup**—Soup made from scratch can be healthy. But overly processed canned soups are packed with sodium, making your blood pressure soar. And while they are convenient, cheap, and fast, canned soups are often not particularly nutrient dense in any one vitamin or mineral.

3. **Processed and fatty meats**—Yes, bacon tastes delicious, and so does a thick, juicy steak. But at a price to your health. Devouring too many fatty cuts of meat like bacon, fatty steaks, sausages, hot dogs, corned beef, fried chicken, and fried fish means loads of unhealthy fat, sodium, and unnecessary calories. Not only do most of these meats contain unhealthy saturated fat, but processing meats often involves salting, curing, or smoking, which raise not only heart disease risk but possibly colorectal cancer risk too. In 2015, the International Agency for Research on Cancer (IARC) classified processed meats as being carcinogenic to humans.[10] In addition, processed meats offer excess calories that usually accumulate as unhealthy belly fat in men.

4. **Alcohol**—No one is saying you can't have your beer, wine, or hard liquor. But if you don't drink in moderation, that is a problem. Drinking in moderation for men is no more than two drinks per day—any more can lead to weight gain and chronic disease. According to the National Institute on Alcohol Abuse and Alcoholism, liver cirrhosis, cancer, pancreatitis, head and neck cancers, high blood pressure, and psychological disorders all are associated with overconsumption of alcohol.

5. **Fast food**—Frequent fast-food stops will knock your intake of sodium, fat, and calories out of the ballpark—but into an unhealthy area. Most fast-food burgers contain 50 to 100 percent of your daily sodium requirements and all of your saturated fat for the day. Excess sodium causes fluid retention and increases blood pressure, while saturated fat spells disaster for increasing your risk of cardiovascular disease. Calorie-wise, a typical quarter-pound

burger with cheese, fries, and soft drink contain 900-plus calories—over 45 percent of a man's daily calorie requirement.

How to Read a Nutrition Facts Label

So, you know you should limit foods high in bad fats, sugar, and salt, while boosting your intake of foods high in healthy fats, fiber, protein, and other nutrients. But how can you decide what's good for you when you're picking out food at the grocery store? A Nutrition Facts label reveals what the food you're eating contains. Not sure what each line means and how to interpret it? Let's break it down for clarification:

Nutrition Facts

About 6 servings per container

Serving size   **1 cup (140g)**

Amount per serving

Calories   170

	% Daily Value*
Total Fat 8g	**10%**
Saturated Fat 3g	**15%**
Trans Fat 0g	
Cholesterol 0mg	**0%**
Sodium 5mg	**0%**
Total Carbohydrate 22g	**8%**
Dietary Fiber 2g	**7%**
Total Sugars 16g	
Includes 8g Added Sugars	**16%**
Protein 2g	
Vitamin D 0mcg	**0%**
Calcium 20mg	**2%**
Iron 1mg	**6%**
Potassium 240mg	**6%**

*The % Daily Value tells you how much a nutrient in a serving of food contributes to a daily diet. 2000 calories a day is used for general nutrition advice.

- **Serving size**—All nutrient amounts shown on the label refer to the serving size. For example, this label shows that the package contains 6 servings, but the serving size (1 cup) is for only 1 serving. So, if you had 2 cups instead of 1 cup, every single number listed below would need to be doubled.

- **Calories**—Want to lose weight? Compare the calories with other similar foods.

- **% daily value**—The daily value is based on nutrient recommendations for a 2,000-calorie diet (indicated at the bottom of the label), but you may need more or less per day. It allows you to compare and evaluate foods' nutrient and calorie contents. A DV of 5 percent or less is considered low. Aim for low saturated fat, trans fat, cholesterol, and sodium. A DV of 20 percent or more is considered high, or a good source of that nutrient. Aim high in vitamins, minerals, and fiber.

- **Saturated fat and trans fat**—To cut your risk of heart disease, look for products with the lowest amount of saturated fat and 0 trans fats per serving.

- **Cholesterol**—Cholesterol guidelines have recently changed, so there is no recommended limit.

- **Sodium**—Choose lower-sodium foods, defined as having no more than 140 mg per serving.

- **Total carbohydrate**—Any food containing sugar, starch, sugar alcohols, and/or fiber will contain carbohydrates.

- **Fiber**—Choose foods with at least 3 grams of fiber per serving.

- **Total sugars**—Total sugars represent sugars found naturally in the food product and sugars that have been added to it.

- **Added sugars**—These are sugars that do not occur naturally in the food and have been added to it, such as brown sugar, molasses, fruit juice concentrate, and high-fructose corn syrup. Choose foods with limited or no added sugars most of the time. Too much sugar can lead to weight gain and can spike blood sugar levels.

What about Dietary Supplements for Men's Health?

Dietary supplements are popular. And surprisingly, men are some of the biggest users of them. According to the Council for Responsible Nutrition 2019 Consumer Survey on Dietary Supplements, the number one reason why 73 percent of all men use a dietary supplement is to improve their overall health/wellness. This same survey also found that of men using a dietary supplement, 78 percent take a multivitamin supplement, 42 percent use an herbal/botanical supplement, and 38 percent use a supplement for enhancing sports nutrition.[11]

But isn't taking a dietary supplement always a positive thing to do? Not in most circumstances. Food should be everyone's first source of nutrients. Eating a balanced diet of real food you can smell, taste, and bite into is the best way to feed your body. Supplements are just that—they were never intended to substitute for food. They cannot replicate all the nutrients and benefits of whole foods, such as fruits and vegetables. Whole foods are complex. They contain a variety of micro-nutrients and protective substances such as antioxidants that help slow down cell and tissue damage. Certain foods also complement one another, packing a bigger nutritional punch known as food synergy. Food synergy is when nutrients in foods work together to create greater health benefits. Dietary supplements won't have this effect; only eating real food does this.

Truth be known, most men who use supplements are already practicing healthy habits of exercising, getting a good night's sleep, watching their weight, not smoking, and trying to eat a healthy diet. More nutrients in supplement form are not necessarily making any further improvements to their health, nor are they a panacea to cure all ailments.

Before using a supplement, you should ask yourself, "Do I really need this, and is it safe?" Let's answer the safety question first. Dietary supplements are under the purview of the U.S. Food and Drug Administration but are regulated differently than conventional foods and drugs. Supplement manufacturers do not have to prove a supplement is safe or that it works before it's sold to the public. But if a supplement is proven to be unsafe after it's been on the market, the FDA can take action to remove or restrict the sale of it.

If you're considering whether to take a dietary or herbal supplement, you should always ask your physician's opinion or, better yet, meet with a registered dietitian to help evaluate your daily diet prior to starting a supplement regimen.

The following charts can guide you in determining whether you need to consider using a supplement. The vast majority are likely unnecessary for most men.

Potential Benefits and Side Effects of Vitamin and Mineral Supplements				
Vitamin or Mineral	RDA for Men	Claim for Taking Supplement	Possible Benefits	Possible Harms
Vitamin D	• 600 IU below age seventy • 800 IU over age seventy-one	• Many adults are deficient, raising risk of chronic illnesses • Few natural dietary sources	• Makes up for low dietary intakes • May reduce risk of prostate cancer and other cancers • Improved bone health	• Kidney or heart damage • Kidney stones • Calcium buildup in blood vessels and soft tissues
Calcium	• 1,000 mg before age seventy • 1,200 mg after age seventy	• Under-consumed nutrient • Deficiency places men at risk of weakened bones and osteoporosis	• Builds and maintains strong bones • May protect from cancer, diabetes, and high blood pressure • Aids in weight loss	• Constipation • Bone pain • Muscle weakness • Reduced absorption of iron and zinc • Kidney stones • Prostate cancer
Vitamin C	• 90 mg, age nineteen and older	• To prevent or treat common colds • To prevent cardiovascular disease, osteroarthritis, and wrinkles	• May reduce length of colds • May reduce risk of stomach, colon, and lung cancers • May slow progression of macular degeneration	• May cause diarrhea, nausea, and stomach cramps • High doses can worsen iron overload and damage body tissue
Vitamin B12	• 2.4 mcg, age nineteen and older	• For older adults and those with digestive tract conditions affecting B12 absorption • To treat a deficiency sometimes found in people following a vegan diet	• To treat or prevent dementia • To control high levels of homocysteine to prevent heart disease • May boost energy and athletic performance	• Body only absorbs what it needs; any excess passes through in urine • Possible interaction with certain medications

Vitamin or Mineral	RDA for Men	Claim for Taking Supplement	Possible Benefits	Possible Harms
Folic acid (synthetic version of natural form of folate found in food)	• 400 mcg, age nineteen and older	• Under-consuming rich food sources such as dark-green leafy vegetables	• Improves heart health • Reduces risk of certain cancers • Reduces depression • Boosts sperm count	• High doses may cause nausea, bloating, gas, and sleep problems • May interfere with some seizure drugs • May mask dangerous lack of vitamin B12
Multi-vitamins		• Convenient • Inexpensive • Backup for a poor diet	• May prevent deficiencies • Few side effects unless taking a megadose	• High doses may increase prostate cancer risk • No evidence they are helpful

Fish Oil Supplements

For years, doctors have recommended fish oil supplements, loaded with omega-3 fatty acids, for protecting against heart disease and stroke, some cancers, arthritis, and more. As mentioned, one of the best sources of omega-3s is fatty fish, which contain DHA and EPA. If you eat fish at least twice a week, you likely will not benefit from extra fish oil.

If you rarely eat fatty fish or nuts and seeds (high in ALA), this is where fish oil supplements may come in. However, before rushing out to buy some, talk to your doctor first. The evidence for fish oil improving heart health is mixed. A 2018 study found that omega-3 fatty acid supplements did nothing to reduce heart attacks, strokes, or deaths from heart disease in middle-aged men without any known risk factors for heart disease.[12] Another 2013 study reported no benefit in people with risk factors for heart disease.[13] But here's the clincher—when researchers looked at subgroups of people who do not eat fish, the results suggested taking a fish oil supplement may reduce their cardiovascular risk after all. The verdict? If your doctor prescribed it, especially for reducing high triglyceride levels, follow their instructions. If you don't eat fish or other seafood, you might benefit from a fish oil supplement, but again, have this discussion with your doctor first.

Selenium Supplements

In 1996, researchers reported that the mineral selenium appeared to reduce the risk of prostate cancer. However, other studies were mixed, raising doubts. Finally, a 2009 multinational trial of selenium and vitamin E supplements, alone or in combination, found that neither nutrient had any benefits against prostate cancer.[14]

Herbal Supplements—Rescue or Risky?

What could go wrong with an herbal supplement? They're all natural and they're used in cooking, so they're relatively harmless, right? Beware. Herbal supplements are often not as safe and reliable as you may think, especially if you have certain medical conditions or take certain medications. Marketers of herbal supplements will tempt you with their magical "cures," but dangers often lurk inside.

Rule number one—if you are using an herbal supplement, you must tell your doctor. When I ask a patient what medications he is taking, I always ask about herbal supplements. That's because the drivers of a man's decision to use herbal supplements often revolve around treating erectile dysfunction or boosting their sex life. But even "natural" remedies can have negative interactions. Here are common herbal supplements you may be using that could have potentially dangerous outcomes:

- **Epimedium, or horny goat weed**—Appropriately named, this herb has been used for years in China for treating sexual dysfunction. It contains a compound called icariin that acts similar to drugs like Viagra. While it may have a beneficial side effect in possibly reducing fatigue and joint pain, the side effects outweigh the good. Nose bleeds, dizziness, rapid heartbeat, and interactions with certain medications should make any man think twice before using this herb.

- **Yohimbe**—Before Viagra and other similar prescription drugs became available, some doctors occasionally prescribed yohimbe for ED as it does promote penile blood flow. This sexual enhancer from South Africa shows some promise in treating impotence. However, concerns have been raised in regard to high blood pressure, anxiety, insomnia, sweating, headaches, and possible heart function damage.

- **Ginseng**—A couple of different forms of ginseng—Panax ginseng and Korean red ginseng—have been used to treat sexual function in men. The belief is that ginseng may work by improving nitric oxide synthesis. The downside of Korean red ginseng in particular is it has not been approved by the FDA for treating ED, and it can interfere with some medications and increase the effects of caffeine.

- **DHEA**—This hormone naturally converts to testosterone and estrogen, helping alleviate some causes of ED. As you know, testosterone is essential for a healthy libido and normal sexual functioning. Because men suffering from ED often have low testosterone, they do show signs of improvement when placed on prescription testosterone replacement therapy. But the over-the-counter DHEA supplement can cause problems like acne, hair loss, and pituitary gland suppression, and the long-term safety is unknown.

- **Ginkgo biloba**—This well-known herbal supplement is commonly used for memory improvement and dementia, but it does not get rave reviews for treating ED, despite many men taking it for this purpose. In fact, most doctors will say this herb doesn't do much. Besides, it can thin your blood, making it especially risky if you take blood-thinning drugs.

Basically, you should always think twice before buying any herbal supplement. In most cases, they are a waste of money and can even threaten your health. Your best bet is to work with your doctor to find beneficial solutions to improve your sexual functioning and your overall health safely. Aside from nutrition, exercise plays a major role in helping accomplish both of these goals, which we'll take a look at next.

SUMMARY

- Men who consistently make healthy food choices over the course of their lifetime are more likely to enjoy good health.

- Adequate daily intakes of both macro- and micronutrients will provide your body with what it needs to perform numerous functions.

- Choosing nutrient-dense foods is key to providing vitamins, minerals, and other beneficial substances with relatively few calories.

- Carbohydrates should be our first choice for adequate energy and fiber. Eating between 30 and 38 grams of fiber daily helps feed our gut microbiome for good gut health, helps lower blood glucose and cholesterol levels, improves weight management, and promotes good colon health.

- Protein is crucial for a variety of bodily functions, from healing wounds to making enzymes, antibodies, and hormones. Food sources of protein are also necessary for the recovery phase of working out and rebuilding muscle afterward. Adding high-quality, lean sources of protein each day is ideal for meeting men's needs.

- Not only does fat make eating pleasurable, but making smart fat choices is valuable for maintaining healthy skin, insulating our body, keeping us feeling fuller longer, and making estrogen and testosterone.

- Certain foods called superfoods are especially healthy for men to consume, such as fatty fish, tart cherries, and tomato sauce, thanks to helping our heart health, reducing oxidative stress, and providing lycopene, a phytochemical good for prostate health.

- All men, regardless of age or activity level, should stay away from not-so-healthy foods such as processed meats, chips, excessive alcohol, and fast food.

- The Nutrition Facts label is a valuable tool you should know how to interpret in order to compare and contrast the best food choices.

- If you think you may need a dietary supplement (vitamins or minerals) or an herbal supplement, you should always discuss this with your primary care physician first to understand the potential benefits and harms.

CHAPTER 10

Movement—Man's Best Friend

Are you a man on the move? Are you exercising, working out, and keeping yourself in good physical condition? Becoming physically fit is a cornerstone of living a long and healthy life. Maybe your life goal is not length of years lived but rather quality of life. If so, perfect. While there are no guarantees how many birthdays you may celebrate, physical activity gives you a stronger, leaner body, with more energy, less chance of age-related diseases, and great sex well into old age. Not bad for a few hours each week of regular, consistent exercise.

Humans are meant to move. Sitting for long stretches at a time hunched over a desk, traveling insanely long work commutes, or reclining every night for endless hours in front of the TV is ruining our health. Never take the ability to move for granted. When we were young and active, running, jumping, climbing trees, and throwing a ball were a given. It felt good to move and to move often. But maybe one day—and maybe that day's already here—bounding out of bed is out of the question due to a stiff, achy body and years of neglecting movement.

Movement is good. Embrace it. When you're physically active, you're sending the message to your brain that you're alive, you're well, you care. But what actually happens to your body when you're moving? Here are a few immediate gratifications you can expect:

Significantly Improves Mood and Attitude

Think of exercise sort of like a happy pill. It's the best natural medicine to chase away the blues, fear, or pain. Here's how: When working out, your brain perceives exercise as stress, putting you into flight-or-fight mode. Your body releases those feel-good hormones called endorphins. As endorphins flood your body, they act as analgesics, interacting with receptors in your brain to reduce your perception of pain. Endorphins are released in response to brain chemicals called neurotransmitters. The neuron receptors endorphins bind to are the same ones that bind with some pain medications. But unlike some addictive pain medications such as morphine, when the body's endorphins activate these receptors, it does not lead to addiction or dependence.

Here's another immediate benefit of exercise—a "runner's high." This is accomplished by another set of neurotransmitters produced in the brain—serotonin and dopamine. Serotonin, which is produced by regular cardiovascular exercise, reduces depression and hostility and improves agreeable behavior.[1] Dopamine improves mood and long-term memory.[2] Both stimulate highly pleasurable feelings in the brain, likely contributing to a positive or euphoric feeling that helps energize and revitalize your outlook on life. Don't care for running? No problem. Even brisk walking, playing tennis, swimming, bicycling, or participating in any other form of movement you enjoy that helps you feel good mentally can produce the same positive effects.

Keeps Muscles from Tightening Up

A special quality of exercise is preventing muscles from becoming overly tight. How do muscles become tight? A common reason is from prolonged periods of inactivity. For example, long days and weeks working seated at a desk can result in tight muscles. When you are seated, your hips are in a bent, or flexed, position. This puts the muscles on the front of the hip (hip flexors) in a shortened position and the muscles on the back of the hips (glutes, or buttocks) in a lengthened position. On top of that, working in front of a computer will put your chest muscles (pectorals) in a shortened position and your upper back muscles (rhomboids) in a lengthened position. Over time, this can result in muscle imbalances, with the shortened muscles becoming "tight" and the lengthened muscles becoming weak. This is why so many people have poor posture with forward, rounded shoulders and underdeveloped glutes. However, keeping mobile with movement, such as taking stretch breaks throughout the day, increases blood flow, taking your muscles from a static state to a very active state. As you move and blood flow increases, it warms up the inactive muscles and releases tightness and soreness from them. This release of tension also allows you to stretch your muscles easier at the end of a workout, which helps lengthen them and restores their optimal function.

Reduces Blood Pressure

Hands down, exercise is a must for lowering blood pressure. With your doctor's approval, cardiovascular workouts such as swimming, bicycling, brisk walking, and jogging can significantly reduce your blood pressure. With age, arteries stiffen, restricting blood flow. Your heart will be working overtime to push blood through inflexible arteries, which causes blood pressure to rise. Exercising releases hormones that help make your blood vessels flexible, which in turn prevents a rise in blood pressure.

Instantly Boosts Your Metabolism

Exercise is the top way to burn calories by increasing your metabolism. The minute you start moving, your heart rate rises, you're breathing more deeply, and your muscles are activated, turning you into a calorie-burning machine. Exercise activates not just your muscles, though—it also activates your brain. Regular movement helps your brain to release neurochemicals that help you burn calories even after your exercise session is done—anywhere from a couple of hours to a couple of days. But to keep your metabolic rate elevated, following a regular routine of consistent exercise is a must.

Taps into Your Creativity

If you find your creative juices have dried up, spend more time exercising. Fitness fanatics will vouch for exercise's effect on brain functioning. Research has found that regular exercise appears to improve creative thinking. From encouraging the growth of new brain cells in the hippocampus to improving memory, even a simple walk can help people come up with new ideas, a mindset that persists even after exercise stops.[3] Regular exercise also appears to improve both divergent and convergent thinking, each considered two components of creative thinking. Divergent thinking involves thinking of multiple solutions for one problem, while convergent thinking involves thinking of one solution for a problem.[4] To really tap into your creative side, take your workout outdoors—spending time in nature boosts cognitive effects too.[5]

Finding the Right Amount of Exercise

While I'm not a personal trainer or exercise physiologist, sometimes I feel like one. Almost every day, I'm asked, "Doc, how much exercise do I need to see health benefits?" This is the kind of million-dollar question that's difficult to answer. Ideally, exercise recommendations should be highly individualized, taking into account your physical abilities, your past health history, and your current health habits and status. It's exactly what I do when asked this common question. My goal is to provide men the best answer for getting and then keeping physically active. It's shocking when you consider that less than a quarter of Americans are meeting all national physical activity guidelines.[6]

I point each man in the right direction by referring and adhering to advice from new guidelines released in November 2018 from the second edition of the *Physical Activity Guidelines for Americans*.[7] These scientifically based guidelines have been researched and recommended by the Department of Health and Human Services and are supported by the American Heart Association. They demonstrate the proven benefits of physical activity, outlining the amount and types of physical activity recommended for different ages and populations.

These recommendations state adults should be aiming for at least 150 minutes a week of moderate-intensity aerobic activity. This can include brisk walking, dancing, bicycling, or jogging. For individuals into more vigorous-intensity aerobic activities, such as running, swimming, or playing tennis or racquetball, 75 minutes each week is the recommendation. Not sure if you are exercising at a moderate or vigorous intensity? Do the "talk test." For moderate-intensity exercise, you should be able to carry on a conversation but not sing. During vigorous exercise, you should be able to say only a few words before needing to take a breath.

The message is any kind of movement or exercise is good, but more is better. However, the reality is for some, finding time to squeeze in a thirty-minute walk or workout at the gym can be daunting. That's why the new guidelines encourage fitting in several five-to-ten-minute sessions throughout the day. Take the stairs and skip the elevator. Walk around when talking on the phone. Conduct walking meetings. Do jumping jacks, knock out some pushups, or jump rope during commercial breaks. Any of these quick and attainable moves makes a difference when added up at the end of the day.

What if you haven't exercised in years? You're not alone—life gets busy, time slips away, and suddenly your six-pack has turned into a keg. (Or maybe you never had a six-pack to begin with!) If you need to gently ease back into exercise or are over the age of sixty-five, start out slowly. Medical professionals recommend using relative intensity rather than absolute intensity as a guide for determining what moderate or vigorous activity is. For example, you should consider how much effort a particular activity takes. Let's say you have a scale from 0 (sitting) to 10 (the most effort required). Moderate-intensity exercise would be defined as a 5 or 6, while vigorous activity would begin at a 7 or an 8. Depending on your fitness level, even tai chi or yoga (usually considered light exercise on an absolute scale) may count as moderate or vigorous activity. Over several weeks or months, gradually build up to a higher intensity and longer session. As you make physical activity a regular part of your lifestyle, even light activity is better than no activity.

It's best to check with your doctor before initiating an exercise program if you are unsteady on your feet, take medications that make you feel dizzy or drowsy, or have a chronic or unstable health condition such as cancer, heart disease, high blood pressure, or diabetes.

The Four Types of Exercise to Include in Your Routine

Exercise is good for everyone. The benefits from even a single bout of activity include improving blood pressure, anxiety, blood sugar, blood cholesterol, sleep, and certain cognitive functions. And consistent exercise has been shown to help reduce cardiovascular disease, type 2 diabetes, dementia, depression, certain cancers, and all-cause mortality. Even bone health is enhanced along with reaching a healthier body image, a healthier body weight, and an overall better quality of life.

Physical activity is not a cure-all, but nearly all people can benefit from increased movement each day, no matter their age, weight, starting fitness level, or health status. I ran across an editorial in the *Journal of the American Medical Association* that summed it up very nicely: "Multiple studies demonstrate that the steepest reduction in disease risk, such as for coronary heart disease, occurs at the lowest levels of physical activity" (that is, from going from no activity to even just a little), and that "reductions in the risk of disease and disability occur by simply getting moving."[8] The most important part of exercise is the fun factor—if you find something you enjoy, it won't even feel like exercise.

So, we know exercise and physical activity is good for us. But what types of exercise should you be including? To be a well-rounded, physically fit person, you need to include the four essential components of physical fitness:

1. Flexibility

2. Muscle strength

3. Muscle endurance

4. Aerobic or cardiorespiratory endurance

If you want to be able to meet the demands of everyday life, you need to work all parts of your body. Think of it like this: if you focused only on jogging but never lifted weights, your aerobic endurance will be great, but your muscle strength will suffer. Or if you work on muscle strength and muscle endurance along with cardio exercise but hardly ever stretch or try to improve flexibility, you'll soon find it difficult just bending over to pick up something from the floor or even getting out of your car without stiffness in your lower back or legs. That's why combining physical activities that work all four areas will be your best bet for achieving a physically fit body.

Flexibility

Out of the four components of physical fitness, flexibility is usually ignored the most by men. However, flexibility is a major part of fitness. Flexibility determines your range of motion—how far you can bend and stretch muscles and ligaments. Without good flexibility, everyday tasks become much harder. No one is saying you have to do the splits with ease, but having too-tight muscles, tendons, and ligaments restricts motion at the joints. If your flexibility is poor, you'll eventually find yourself in a predicament of not easily bending over to tie your shoes, striding out when walking, or stretching to remove packages from your car. Improving flexibility also reduces your risk of injuries, such as pulled muscles and strained tendons when exercising.

Only ten to fifteen minutes a day of stretching will significantly improve flexibility, enhancing your ability to move with ease. No idea on how to become more flexible? That's okay—here are some of the best stretches to work your whole body. Perform each one on both sides, on a mat if you prefer, ideally one to five sets for fifteen to thirty seconds each day:

Quad stretch

Stretches the quadriceps muscles, the large muscle in front of the thigh.

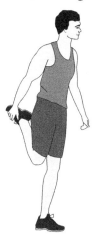

Stand upright and bend one leg back, grabbing the top of that foot. Bring your foot as close to your butt as possible while keeping your bent knee in line with your other knee. Push your hips forward for a deepened stretch. Hold on to a wall for balance if needed. Repeat with the other leg.

Standing hamstring stretch

Stretches the back of the thighs, keeping these muscles loose and flexible; improves posture and reduces lower back pain.

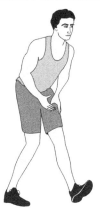

Stand upright, bending one knee and extending the other out straight in front of you about six inches, heel on the ground and toes pointing up. Bend at the hips, keeping your back straight. Lower your chest until you feel a stretch in the back of the extended leg, and hold for up to 10 seconds or more. Repeat with the other leg.

Inner thigh stretch

Improves flexibility in the quadriceps and hip flexors;
relieves tension in the lower back and hips.

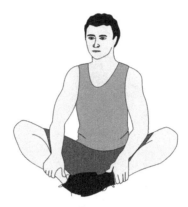

Sit up straight on the ground with knees bent so that the soles of your feet touch one another. Grasp your feet with your hands. Gently push down on your knees with your elbows to deepen the stretch.

"Eye of the needle" stretch

Relieves discomfort; decreases tightness and increases hip mobility.

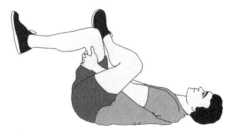

Lie on your back with knees bent and feet flat on the floor. Hug your left knee into your chest. Place your left ankle onto the right thigh. Lift your right foot up and then thread your left hand through your legs so both hands meet on the back side of your right thigh. Use your hands to draw your right thigh toward your chest while exhaling and keeping both feet flexed. Return to the starting position and repeat on the other side.

Chest and shoulder stretch

Increases flexibility and range of motion in the chest and provides pain-free movement of the shoulders to help improve upper body posture.

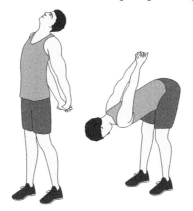

Stand up straight or sit on a surface so that your legs are at a 90-degree angle. Clasp your hands together behind your back so that your arms are extended behind you. Lift your hands to the ceiling to stretch your chest and shoulders. Then, bend forward at the hips with your head pointed toward your feet with your clasped hands reaching toward the ceiling. Return to the starting position and repeat.

Half-kneeling hip flexor stretch

Stretches hip flexors, which is important for people who sit most of the day.

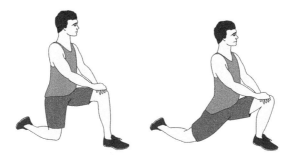

Lower yourself onto your knees. Lift your left knee so it's bent at a 90-degree angle, and plant your left foot on the floor. Exhale and lean forward until you feel the stretch in your upper thigh and hip flexors. Your left knee should never go beyond your toes. Your right knee and toes should stay on the floor during the entire stretch. Hold the stretch for thirty seconds. Return to the starting position and repeat on the other side.

Hamstring walkouts

*Targets your hamstrings, calves, and lower back,
improving flexibility and blood flow.*

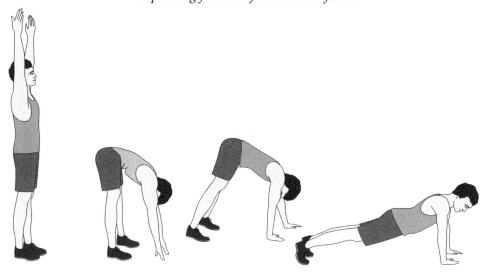

While standing, hinge at your hips and reach down toward your toes until you touch the floor, keeping your legs straight. If you can't reach the floor, bend your knees so you can. As soon as your hands touch the floor, alternately walk them forward until you're in a pushup position. Your legs should be straight and at the same height as your head, shoulders, and hips. Begin to walk your hands back toward your feet while pushing your hips in the air, driving your heels into the floor (sort of like mimicking an inchworm). Keep your legs straight as long as you can to get a good stretch. Return to a standing position and repeat nine times.

Standing side bend

Warms up and preps the serratus muscle (a muscle around your ribcage).

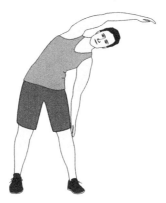

Stand with your feet hip-width apart. Raise your left hand up and over your head and keep your right hand by your side. Engage your abdominals (imagine pulling your belly button in toward your spine) and bend at the waist toward your right side, lowering your right arm toward the floor as you go. Hold for a few seconds, then slowly return to the starting position. Repeat on the other side. Complete ten reps on each side.

Happy baby pose

Opens the hips, stretches the inner groin, decompresses and lengthens the spine, calms the mind, and relieves stress.

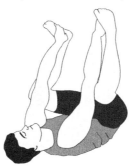

Lie on your back. With an exhale, bend your knees into your belly. Inhaling, grip the outsides of your feet with your hands. Open your knees slightly wider than your torso, then bring them up toward your armpits. Position each ankle directly over the knee, so your shins are perpendicular to the floor. Flex through the heels. Gently push your feet up into your hands as you pull your hands down to create resistance. Hold for a minimum of ten breaths. The longer you hold, the better the stretch.

Child's pose

Helps stretch the hips, thighs, and ankles while reducing stress and fatigue.

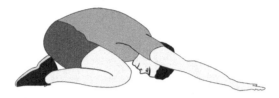

Start in a kneeling position. Drop your butt toward your heels as you stretch the rest of your body down and forward. In the fully stretched position, rest your arms in a relaxed position along the floor, rest your stomach comfortably on top of your thighs, and rest your forehead on the mat. You should feel a mild stretch in your shoulders and buttocks and down the length of your spine and arms.

Bird-dog stretch

Strengthens the core muscles, specifically the abdominals, lower back, butt, and thighs.

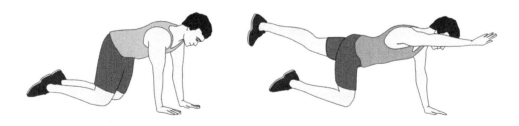

Begin on your hands and knees in the tabletop position, placing your knees under your hips and your hands under your shoulders. Maintain a neutral (flat) spine by engaging your abdominal muscles. Raise your right arm and left leg, keeping your shoulders and hips parallel to the floor. Lengthen the back of your neck and tuck your chin into your chest to gaze down at the floor. Hold this position for a few seconds, and then lower back down to the starting position. Raise your left arm and right leg, holding this position for a few seconds. Return to the starting position. Do two to three sets of eight to twelve repetitions.

Muscle Strength and Muscle Endurance

As men, if we want to grow old gracefully, we must maintain muscle strength and muscle endurance. That's why every day you should do physical activities that enhance both. In case you're wondering what the difference is between muscle strength and muscle endurance, let me explain.

Muscle strength is what enhances your ability to perform tasks such as lifting or pushing. If you fail to maintain muscle strength, your ability to lift a gallon of milk off the top shelf of the refrigerator with one hand, carry the trash to the curb, or move a couch into your living room will be very difficult if not impossible as you age.

Muscle endurance is your ability to continue repetitive muscle activity, such as shoveling snow or raking leaves. If you were a competitive athlete in long-distance running during high school or college or ever competed in a triathlon, you had or may still have great muscle endurance.

Every day we perform tasks that require muscle use: pulling a heavy suitcase, carrying a bag of groceries, and prying open a box that's taped shut all depend on our muscles. Increasing both muscle strength and muscle endurance is contingent on repeatedly using our muscles in activities that require moving against resistance. This type of exercise is called muscle-strengthening exercise, or resistance-training exercise. One of the best examples of meeting this need is weight training, or weight lifting. Weight lifting stresses the muscles, causing them to adapt by increasing their size and strength—a process called hypertrophy. The larger, stronger muscles can lift the same weight more easily. Muscles that are not used due to a lapse in weight training, injury, or illness become smaller and weaker. This process is called atrophy. So, you can see why there is truth to the saying, "Use it or lose it."

If you're already actively engaged in strength and endurance training by using weights or machines at a gym, or if you work with a personal trainer, keep doing so. If it's been awhile since you've lifted weights, start off slowly and gradually. Some moves such as pushups or pull-ups require only your body weight to help strengthen and build muscle. Otherwise, a few pairs of dumbbells of different weights can help build muscle, burn calories, and enhance cardiovascular fitness. Here are a few examples of how to get started lifting weights at home:

Goblet squat

Targets glute activation while improving both hip and thoracic mobility.

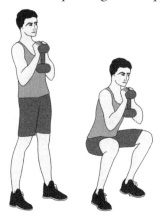

Stand with feet set wider than shoulder-width apart and hold a dumbbell with both hands in front of your chest. Sit back into a deep squat position, keeping your knees aligned with your toes, and then press back up through your heels, exhaling as you rise while pressing your hips forward at the top of the squat, fully engaging your glutes. Complete a set of five reps, and aim for a total of three to five sets or more.

Bent-over row

Targets the trapezoid, rhomboids, laterals, and biceps; perfect for getting that "V" shape.

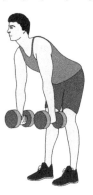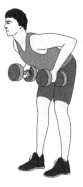

With legs slightly bent and your core tight and back straight, bend by pushing your hips backward until your upper body is almost perpendicular to the floor. Row the weights (either dumbbells or a barbell) up to the lower part of your chest. Pause, slowly lower to a count of five, and repeat: do eight to twelve repetitions for each arm, rest for two minutes, then do another set per arm.

One-arm swing

With proper form, builds grip strength, coordination,
lower back muscles, quadriceps, and shoulders.

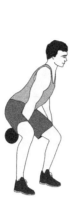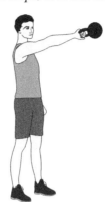

Stand with feet shoulder-width apart and knees slightly bent. Hold a dumbbell or kettlebell in one hand, sink into a squat, and swing the dumbbell through your legs. Immediately drive yourself forward, bringing the weight upward and forward while squeezing your glutes. Repeat this movement with eight to twelve repetitions, and then change hands. Rest for two minutes, then do another set per arm.

Bench press with dumbbells

Works the pectoral, back, and shoulder muscles.

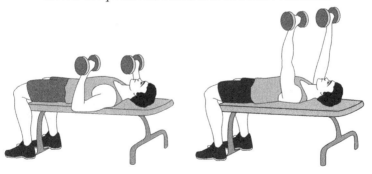

Lie face up on a flat bench with your feet planted flat on the floor, holding a dumbbell in each hand just outside your shoulders. Bend your elbows at roughly 90 degrees, pointed out and just under your torso. Holding each dumbbell with your palms facing toward your feet, powerfully press the dumbbells toward the ceiling by flexing your pecs and extending your elbows, stopping when the inner plates of the weights are an inch or so away from each other. Then slowly return the dumbbells to the starting position. Do eight to twelve repetitions, rest, then do another set.

Cross-body hammer curl

By focusing on one arm at a time, engages the nervous system to recruit more muscle fibers.

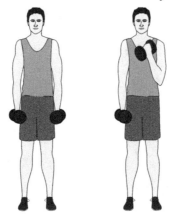

Standing up straight, hold a dumbbell in each hand with palms facing inward. One at a time, curl each weight up toward your opposing shoulder, isolating the bicep and squeezing the muscle. Hold for one count. Return slowly back to starting position and repeat on the other side.

Step-ups

Fires up your gluteus maximus, the major muscle responsible for extending, rotating, and adducting and abducting from the hip joint.

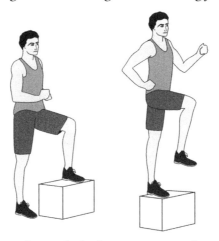

Place your left foot onto an elevated platform, or step and push up through your heel to lift yourself up and then place your right foot on the platform. Step back down with your right foot and then the left. Repeat on the other side. Do eight to twelve repetitions per leg of two sets. For more resistance, hold a dumbbell in each hand.

Lateral raises

Targets the deltoid muscles; can ward off potential injuries if done regularly as the shoulder is the least stable joint in the body; gives the appearance of broader, stronger shoulders.

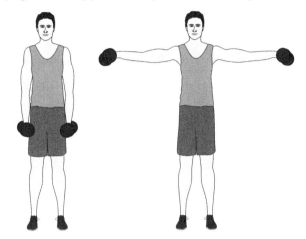

Stand tall, positioning your feet hip-distance apart, and hold a dumbbell in each hand at your sides, palms facing in. Check your posture by rolling your shoulders back and in, engage your core, and look straight ahead. Keeping your elbows slightly bent, raise your arms straight out to the sides until they're at shoulder level. Pause, then slowly lower the weights back to the starting position. Focus on moving in a slow, controlled fashion with each rep. Do eight to twelve repetitions, rest, then do another set.

Strength and balance

Strength training also helps improve balance. Poor balance increases the risk of dangerous falls often due to loss of muscle strength and joint flexibility, as well as reduced vision and reaction time. Achieving and having good balance is a complex feat involving various sensory and motor systems, including vision (to perceive direction and motion), the vestibular system in the inner ear, and another important component called *proprioception*, or the ability to sense where your body is within its space. Just the ability to remain steady on your feet requires good muscle strength and reaction time.

Even if you are a naturally agile person, everyone needs to work on balance as they age. Just like maintaining your muscle strength or flexibility, balance must be challenged through specific techniques that keep you steady on your feet. Here are a few simple balancing tips you can do just about anywhere.

On-the-Go Balance Training

- Practice standing on one leg while brushing your teeth, cooking, showering, or combing your hair.

- Stand on one leg for ten to fifteen seconds, then switch legs; repeat ten times. Then do it again with your eyes closed.

- Pick up objects (newspaper, shoes, pen, etc.) while standing on one leg.

- Walk heel to toe. Take twenty steps forward heel to toe, then walk backward with toe to heel in a straight line.

- Without holding on to anything, rise up on your toes ten times. Repeat with your eyes closed.

- Stand on one foot with hands on hips, and place your nonsupporting foot against the inside of the knee of your standing leg. Raise your heel off the floor, and hold the pose for up to twenty-five seconds. Repeat on the other side.

- Stand with feet together, anklebones touching and arms folded across your chest. Close your eyes and time yourself for sixty seconds without moving your feet. Then place one foot directly in front of the other and close your eyes, standing for up to thirty seconds on each foot.

Aerobic or Cardiorespiratory Endurance

If you're like me and like to bicycle, play tennis, or go on a brisk walk, you'll need good cardiorespiratory endurance. Imagine you're exercising, working up a sweat. You're breathing hard, your heart is beating faster, and blood is coursing through your vessels, delivering oxygen to your muscles and keeping you moving. You are doing what is known as aerobic exercise.

The word *aerobic*, or "with oxygen," means more oxygen-carrying blood is circulating throughout your tissues and being delivered to your working muscles. Accomplishing this action requires an increase in heart rate and stroke volume, which is the amount of blood pumped by the heart with each heartbeat.

To really get a good idea of your aerobic or cardiorespiratory fitness, you would need to measure the maximum amount of oxygen your muscles consume during exercise, or VO_2max. If you're a very physically fit person, you will have a higher VO_2max with the ability to exercise at a higher intensity without fatigue than someone who is not as fit.

All of us should focus on improving our aerobic or cardiorespiratory fitness. With heart disease as the leading cause of death in the US, it's a must for lowering your risk of this malady. Aerobic exercise is ideal for lowering heart rate, blood pressure, cholesterol, and stress levels, and it aids in weight loss.

Fortunately, there are many forms of aerobic activity. Examples include running, bicycling, swimming, walking, hiking, dancing, cross-country skiing, and kickboxing. Find at least one type (or more) of aerobic exercise you enjoy doing. If you like it, you're more likely to stick with it long term.

Here are other smart reasons aerobic exercise, along with flexibility, muscle strength, and muscle endurance activities, needs to be part of your fitness regimen:

The Benefits of Physical Fitness	
Benefit	**How It Works**
Reduced risk of heart disease	Research shows that moderate physical activity lowers blood pressure[9] and is positively associated with HDL (good) cholesterol.[10]
Improved body composition	Exercise helps burn excess stored body fat and builds muscle, resulting in a leaner body mass. Those who participate in aerobic fitness have less total fat and abdominal fat compared with people who don't participate in aerobic fitness often or at all.[11]
Reduced risk of type 2 diabetes	Exercise helps control blood glucose levels by increasing insulin sensitivity.[12]
Reduced risk of some forms of cancer	Increased physical activity has been associated with a reduced risk of colon, breast, endometrial, and lung cancers.[13]
Improved bone health	Bone density has been shown to improve with weight-bearing exercise and resistance training, reducing the risk of osteoporosis.[14]
Improved immune system	Regular moderate exercise can enhance the immune system by increasing immunoglobulins in the body, which protect against colds and other infectious diseases.[15]
Improved mental well-being	Regular exercise protects against onset of depression and anxiety disorders.[16]
Improved sleep	People who exercise regularly often have better-quality sleep due to reduced anxiety, antidepressant effects, and body temperature changes that promote sleep.[17]

SUMMARY

- A cornerstone of good health is keeping yourself physically fit.

- Prolonged periods of inactivity can result in various health conditions.

- Physical activity can have immediate benefits such as improving mood, reducing muscle tightness, lowering blood pressure, increasing metabolism to burn off excess calories, and enhancing brain activity.

- Official exercise guidelines recommend at least 150 minutes a week of moderate-intensity aerobic activity or 75 minutes of vigorous aerobic activity.

- To become a well-rounded, physically fit person, you need to practice the four essential components of physical fitness—flexibility, muscle strength, muscle endurance, and aerobic or cardiorespiratory endurance.

- Flexibility is crucial for maintaining range of motion and making everyday tasks easier.

- Muscle strength is necessary to perform tasks such as lifting or pushing, while muscle endurance enhances your ability to do repetitive muscle activity for a certain length of time.

- Aerobic or cardiorespiratory endurance delivers many health benefits, from lowered blood pressure to increased heart strength. Examples include brisk walking, swimming, and dancing.

CHAPTER 11

Man's Dual Nemesis—Lack of Sleep and Stress Overload

Bad sleep and stress—talk about a double-edged sword. When men lack sleep, our stress levels rise, and when stress levels rise, we lack sleep. Each of us has felt the brunt of stress and know its powerfully brutal grip affects all aspects of life, especially sleep.

Since stress never completely goes away and since sleep is a necessity for good health, this chapter is devoted to helping you find the right balance of each. I particularly want you to avoid this conversation with yourself when you're trying to get some sleep:

You: "I want to fall asleep."

Your brain: "Not me. I'm working overdrive, going over every single problem in your life that's bothering you."

You: "Okay, if you insist, but I'd really rather sleep."

Talk about a stressful conversation. If you've found yourself with these thoughts when trying to fall asleep, this chapter is for you. When you're struggling with stress and lack of sleep, thinking through your problems at bedtime only exacerbates the situation. Once you learn how to get a good night's sleep and deal more effectively with stressful situations, you'll have conquered a huge troublesome dynamic of your life, setting you on the road to better health and happiness.

Sleep—Your Most Valuable Activity of the Day

If you were to ask any man about his priorities for the day, you'd probably never hear him mention getting healthy sleep. Many men view sleep as wasted time that prevents them from getting work done. This is not a wise viewpoint. Insufficient sleep is often a common obstacle that keeps men from tapping into the power of a well-rested mind and body. Men who invest in sufficient sleep will see a bigger return in everything else they do. Night after night of good sleep enables you to think, feel, and perform better. You'll do a better job maximizing your time and energy during the day all because you're giving your body the sleep it needs.

Besides, quality shut-eye also helps you handle stress and improves your overall well-being. Sleep is your body's time to heal, recharge, and restore itself. Skimp on it, and that sleep debt affects every aspect of your daily functioning and health, from your memory to your mood to the number of sick days you take to even your risk for a heart attack. Sufficient sleep is that important.

How Lack of Sleep Affects Your Health

Who hasn't heard from their doctor these words: "Eat a healthy diet and get plenty of exercise"? It's good advice for all men. However, even if you're doing that but lack sleep, you may be undermining those efforts. So, how much sleep do you need? This was answered in a 2015 issue of the National Sleep Foundation's journal *Sleep Health*, which provides updates on sleep recommendations. These recommendations are broken down into age-specific categories with a time range for each, allowing for individual differences[1]:

- Older adults, sixty-five and up: seven to eight hours
- Adults, twenty-six to sixty-four: seven to nine hours
- Young adults, eighteen to twenty-five: seven to nine hours

Of course, depending on your genetics, behavioral and environmental factors will help determine how much sleep you require for your best health and daily performance.

When you short yourself on shut-eye, it has a negative impact on your short-term health:

- Lack of alertness
- Impaired memory
- Relationship stress
- Poorer quality of life
- Greater likelihood for car accidents

Chronic sleep deprivation can even affect your appearance, leading to premature wrinkles and dark circles and bags under your eyes.

Why Adequate Sleep Is Your Best Medicine

If you've never considered sleep one of your biggest health assets, it's time you should. In case you need more convincing, here is how sleep plays a major role in your health:

- **Boosts heart health**—Poor sleep quality is linked to heart health problems such as high blood pressure and heart attacks. Shortchanging yourself on sleep can lead to a surge in stress hormones like cortisol. Stress is a normal part of life, but constant, long-term stress can increase blood cholesterol, triglycerides, blood sugar, and blood pressure, all risk factors for heart disease. It also promotes plaque buildup in arteries, increasing the risk of stroke and heart attack.

- **Prevents packing on pounds**—Looking to drop a few pounds? Get a good night's sleep. Research suggests an association between sleep restriction and negative changes in metabolism. In adults, sleeping only four hours a night compared to ten hours can increase hunger and appetite—especially for calorie-dense foods high in carbohydrates.[2] Sleeplessness cranks up production of the hormone ghrelin, which boosts appetite, and reduces production of the hormone leptin, which signals feeling full. When you're stressed, lack energy, and are sleep deprived, it's a perfect storm for craving junk food. Give in to the office vending machine, and that candy bar will send your blood sugar surging, then crashing, leaving your appetite raging all over again.

- **Strengthens your immune system**—High-quality rest keeps your immune cells and immune system proteins in fighting shape to help you resist colds, the flu, and other infections.

- **Improves brain health**—Your brain on sleep deprivation is not a pretty sight. Too many sleepless nights sets you up for unclear thinking, an inability to focus, and difficulty in memory recall. This can lead to potentially disastrous mistakes at work or at home. Proper sleep is linked to improved concentration and higher cognitive functioning.

- **Fires up your sex life**—Being too exhausted for sex is no way to live. But when you lack quality shut-eye, your testosterone levels can suffer. Men who sleep less than six hours nightly have lower levels of testosterone, which can quickly sink your sex life since low levels of this hormone can result in erectile dysfunction.

- **Decreases number of headaches**—A common headache trigger is inadequate sleep. People living with headaches have almost twice the rates of insomnia as those with infrequent headaches. A good start to reducing headaches is to get regular sleep.

- **Boosts your mood**—Getting a well-rested night of sleep makes you wake up feeling optimistic. You have more energy and drive, and you're less likely to let small challenges such as a heavy workload or heavy traffic lead to frustration or anger. Sleepless nights will only make you cranky, irritable, and more vulnerable to stress and anxiety.

The Six Biggest Factors Preventing Men from Getting Enough Sleep

There are several common reasons men are sleep deprived. Chances are at least one of these applies to you:

1. Work Demands

Men often have time-demanding jobs, leaving little room for adequate sleep. In order to get ahead, you might put in those extra hours, work on the weekends, or be the first person who shows up to work. Add in a long commute through heavy traffic, and even more hours of the day are taken up without sleep. Even when you're finally home, your work still consumes your time. There may be paperwork to finish, emails to answer, a cell phone that won't stop ringing. Before you know it, it's another late night working way past your bedtime.

Demanding, stressful jobs affect sleep. Worry, doubt, and anxiety may take over your mind when your head hits the pillow, and when your mind is spinning, your body will have difficulty winding down and falling asleep. This leads to another night tossing and turning or staring at the clock ticking away until the alarm goes off.

What to do—Start by leaving your work responsibilities at work. Your body and mind need a break with rest and relaxation away from work duties. Setting boundaries is important as your personal time is valuable. If you work from home, find ways to get out of the house to relax and unwind. Talking with your spouse or a good friend who will listen helps to relieve pent-up stress. Exercising regularly to help release tension and the feel-good endorphins will make you feel better physically and mentally. Most of all, remember your bed is a place of rest and pleasure, not worry.

2. Lack of Awareness of Sleep Deprivation

If you've ever been asked if you feel tired, it's likely you answered, "Always." If not, you've probably heard another man express that he's chronically exhausted. When we're used to feeling tired, we may assume it's because we are working hard, and that's just the way it is. Besides, fighting through that feeling gives us more time to work. However, most adults need on average seven to eight hours of sleep each night just to feel alert and well rested. Most men aren't consistently meeting that need, though, preventing us from functioning at a maximum level of energy and concentration.

How do you know if you are not getting enough sleep? Here are some clues:

- Feeling tired and lacking energy during the day
- Having trouble paying attention at work or during meetings
- Feeling unmotivated
- Being irritable, grouchy, and easily angered
- Always using an alarm clock to wake up
- Feeling sleepy while driving

What to do—It may sound obvious, but start by going to bed earlier. Plan to go to bed early enough to allow yourself at least seven to eight hours before you need to wake up in the morning. Eliminate all caffeine at least six hours or more before bedtime and all fluid intake at least two hours before. Take a warm shower and stretch to relax your muscles and mind. Make love with your partner—that's always a perfect way to end the day.

3. Too Many Activities

Our worst enemy snatching away time from sleep is an overscheduled life. On the one hand, it's good to be involved, whether it's volunteer work, family time, hobbies, working out, or belonging to an organization. All benefit you in various ways. But if the list of people, places, and things to do is leaving you exhausted, something has got to give.

What to do—Set priorities to learn to balance your time. Decide what you enjoy doing and what you could live without. If being on a certain committee is taking up valuable time, consider going off it and joining back up in the future. It's okay to scale back, especially if it's not a high priority. Remember, sleep is a high priority, so make it an activity of importance.

4. Lifestyle Changes

It's guaranteed—whether positive or negative, life is always changing. Positive changes lead to a richer, fuller life—getting married, having a baby, starting a new job, or moving. Negative changes, however, can keep you up at night—losing a loved one, losing a job, getting divorced, getting diagnosed with a major illness, being in a car wreck. The not-so-welcomed changes can lead to feelings of despair and depression. Not only is your sleep disrupted, but you may also lack motivation to get out of bed. Poor sleep often leads to neglecting healthy habits too—you may stop exercising, abuse alcohol or drugs, and lose interest and pleasure in normal activities of daily life.

What to do—One of our worst qualities as men is resisting help when we need it. We have to understand it's perfectly normal to have negative feelings; we just can't ignore them or let them overtake our health. If you're overwhelmed by negative changes in your life, start by talking to your spouse or partner, friends, doctor, spiritual leader, or mental health counselor. Don't fight this battle alone.

5. Bad Habits Affecting Sleep

Alcohol, nicotine, caffeine, and big meals are all sleep-disrupting habits. Do them too close to bedtime and you will likely experience a restless night. Maintaining an irregular sleep schedule can also cause problems falling and staying asleep.

What to do—Simple solutions include avoiding alcohol and caffeine several hours before bedtime, quitting smoking, eating a bigger lunch and a smaller dinner, and going to bed and waking up at the same times each day. Your body's internal clock likes a regular sleep-wake pattern, even on weekends and holidays. On days you feel tired, though, go to bed earlier. If you take a nap, do so early in the afternoon for no more than thirty minutes.

6. Medical Conditions

Whether it's the flu, a sprained ankle, arthritis, or another chronic health ailment, many medical conditions can keep you up at night. Unfortunately, as you get older, health conditions become more common. Even medications used to treat health problems can hinder you from getting quality sleep.

What to do—If the condition is temporary, you may have to adjust by getting more rest during the day and keeping yourself as comfortable as possible while sleeping. If medications for a chronic condition are causing side effects like jitteriness or excessive sleepiness during the day, have a discussion with your doctor. See if the dose or when you take the drug can be changed to allow for more restful sleep.

If sleepless nights or excessive tiredness during the day is due to obstructive sleep apnea or narcolepsy, you should see a sleep specialist to get an accurate diagnosis and the best treatment method for your situation.

How Men Can Improve Sleep Hygiene

Getting a restful night of sleep begins with developing good sleep hygiene habits. Sleep hygiene includes different practices and habits necessary to have good nighttime sleep quality and full daytime alertness. When practiced regularly, these habits can make a world of difference in how you feel, look, and perform on the job and at home. You'll see that we've already touched on a few of them.

Good Sleep Hygiene Practices

- Limit daytime naps to no more than thirty minutes.
- Avoid stimulants such as caffeine and nicotine close to bedtime.
- Exercise to promote good-quality sleep.
- Steer clear of heavy or rich foods, fatty or fried meals, spicy dishes, citrus fruits, and carbonated beverages right before sleep as they can trigger indigestion and heartburn.
- Get adequate exposure to natural light during the day, which helps maintain a healthy sleep-wake cycle.
- Establish a regular, relaxing bedtime routine that might include a warm shower or bath, reading a book, or light stretches.
- Create a pleasant sleep environment—sleep on a comfortable mattress and pillows, keep the bedroom cool at 60 to 67 degrees, and power down from all electronics (cell phones, computers, tablets, laptops, and TV screens). Consider using blackout curtains, eyeshades, earplugs, white noise such as a fan, and other devices that make the bedroom more relaxing.

Source: Sleepfoundation.org

The Effect of Stress on Men's Health

Think you're invincible to stress? How well did you handle yesterday's rush-hour traffic that made you arrive home forty-five minutes late? Or how often does your boss or coworker cause you to mumble *blankety-blank* under your breath? How about how you handled the recent computer glitch that wasted valuable time on an important project? Admit it: our modern-day world has become extremely stressful. So stressful that back in 2015, a survey by the American Psychological Association found that average stress levels in the US rose from 4.9 in 2014 to 5.1 in 2015 on a 10-point scale. That same year, 24 percent of those surveyed reported they experienced more stress than in the previous year, compared with 18 percent in 2014.[3] However, the 2020 COVID-19 pandemic ranked extremely high as the most stressful time in American history, affecting every single person from the young to the elderly. Record unemployment, school closings, lockdowns, social distancing, and high mortality rates all led to high anxiety, uncertainty, and depression among both men and women.[4]

Every day, you will deal with some sort of stress. It's unavoidable. However, not all stress is considered bad. Good stress might be watching the birth of your child or going out on a first date. The not-so-good stresses of life can range from minor situations such as arguing with your spouse or getting stuck in traffic to more major stresses such as getting a cancer diagnosis or experiencing the death of a loved one.

Everyone responds to stress in their own way. We already recognized that many of us respond poorly by trying to address our stress at bedtime. But if stress hangs like a dark cloud casting its shadow over your life, or if it continually comes to a boiling point, your health and quality of life will be negatively affected sooner than later. Those nagging headaches, insomnia, or reduced productivity at work may actually be due to constant stress.

Our fast-paced, modern age of technology makes us struggle to keep up with day-to-day responsibilities, bringing tension and strain that may lead to chronic health conditions like heart disease, high blood pressure, diabetes, cancer, and a weakened immune system. Even short-term stress can heighten anxiety, insomnia, fatigue, and depression—as well as contribute to ED, which you may recall from an earlier chapter. Men under stress may react by resorting to unhealthy habits like drinking too much, smoking, overeating, or using illegal drugs.

How to Turn Down Your Body's Stress Volume

In earlier eras, stress was a far cry from the stress of today. Wild animals would chase a man seeking food for his family, triggering his fight-or-flight response. This response prompted certain physical changes within his body to get him out of the tough situation.

Today, our body under stress still resorts to that same response, except we no longer are running from wild animals—we are trying to meet a deadline or worrying over financial concerns. But our physical response is still the same:

- Increased heart rate, sending more blood to the brain to improve quick thinking
- More blood flow to large muscles of the legs and arms, providing strength and speed
- Increased blood sugar, providing quick energy
- Blood clotting more quickly after a wound or an injury, preventing blood loss

These responses are great when you need to fight or flee but not necessarily when you simply need to relax and reduce anxiety. The next time you feel stress bearing down on you, here are some simple ways to reduce its toxic effects:

1. **Eat a healthy diet.** Nutrition and stress are interlinked; feed your body poorly, and it'll become one of your biggest enemies by increasing your risk of future health problems, particularly when dealing with stress. Instead, make food your greatest ally by choosing health-promoting foods to help counter the impact of stress. Consume more fruits, vegetables, legumes, and whole grains while cutting back on refined, processed foods. Don't resort to overeating junk, which puts on pounds.

2. **Exercise regularly.** There is nothing like exercise for burning off pent-up energy, tension, and anxiety.

3. **Get adequate sleep.** As mentioned, keep a regular bedtime and avoid caffeine and alcohol several hours before turning in to prevent sleep interruptions, sleeplessness, and anxiety.

4. **Avoid stressful situations.** This is easier said than done, but it's very effective advice. For example, if rush hour is your stress trigger, avoid it by driving a different route. Can't stand certain people who stress you out? Avoid them as much as possible.

5. **Figure out the cause of your stress.** Most men like to figure out solutions to problems, so when we deal with the root cause—whatever is creating the tension, in this case—we can usually address it successfully.

6. **Meditate.** You may not consider meditation manly or a good use of time, but just the simple act of closing your eyes in quiet contemplation for five to ten minutes can bring about peace and clear your mind.

7. **Avoid taking on too many tasks.** Overscheduling and always saying yes to others can take its toll. Avoid overpromising, and allow time to complete what you start before accepting anything else.

8. **Learn to tackle first things first.** Men are usually very good at this, but sometimes if we have too many tasks to tackle, it can be stressful. Start with the most important task, and then move on to less critical tasks that can wait.

9. **Take time off for some fun.** Everyone needs a break from the same stressful routine, and what better way to burn off steam than by doing something fun? Taking time to do what we enjoy calms us down and fosters a sense of relaxation, spontaneity, and well-being.

10. **Listen to music.** Specific kinds of music like classical music can have measurable stress-reducing effects for many people. This effect can make you feel more centered and reduce anxiety, depression, and stress-inducing cortisol levels.

11. **Laugh a little—or a lot.** A good belly laugh can have impressive short-term effects—it stimulates your heart, lungs, and muscles (by enhancing your intake of oxygen-rich air) and increases endorphins released by the brain. Laughter also temporarily fires up your stress response by increasing your heart rate and blood pressure, so you feel relaxed as soon as the response cools down. Having a good sense of humor can also improve immune function, relieve pain, improve mood, and reduce anxiety and depression.

12. **Learn to see the big picture of life.** No one gets through life without having ups and downs—no one. When we consider what is stressing us out by asking ourselves, "How can I see this situation in a different way?" it can remind us that life ebbs and flows, and there is always someone out there who has it much worse. Better times will return, and getting through tough times only makes us stronger in the long run.

Now that sleep and stress have been covered, it's time to turn our attention in the last chapter of this book to one of men's greatest enjoyments—food.

SUMMARY

- Sufficient, quality sleep is necessary for improving energy, stress levels, immune functioning, and overall quality of life.

- Sleep improves heart and brain health, helps you maintain a healthy body weight, and can boost your sex life.

- Many factors prevent men from getting enough sleep. Use strategies such as prioritizing your tasks and exercising regularly to overcome these obstacles.

- Practice good sleep hygiene for better sleep.

- Stress affects everyone. Part of men's health may depend on how much stress they experience and how they respond to it.

- Devise a plan on how to defuse stress to help prevent its toxic effects.

PART 4

Nutritious, Hearty Recipes for Meal Planning

CHAPTER 12

Delicious Recipes
for Keeping Men Healthy

Next to sex and back rubs, good food will keep many a man happy and satisfied. Without question, men love to eat. There's nothing wrong with that. However, promoting and protecting our health in the best way possible begins with choosing food that's nourishing but also tastes great. Let's be realistic—it could be the healthiest food the universe has seen, but if it tastes disgusting, there's no way anyone will want to eat it. This chapter has twenty-four delicious recipes that focus on nutritional value and why and how each one is good for men. The recipes were chosen based on their appeal to men, simplicity and ease of assembly, and most of all, taste. All the recipes use easy-to-find ingredients and are perfectly doable as an early morning breakfast, a quick lunch, or a weeknight meal. My own Mediterranean Salmon (page 200) is a personal favorite I've enjoyed many times with my family and friends, and I hope you will like it too. Each recipe provides fresh ingredients of fruits, vegetables, lean beef, fish and chicken, nuts, low-fat dairy, and whole grains that easily meet dietary standards for good heart, prostate, and brain health.

Before we get to the recipes, let's talk about tuning up the most important room in your home for achieving great health—the kitchen.

Stocking a Healthy Kitchen

Getting healthy begins in the kitchen. When your pantry, refrigerator, and freezer are well stocked with nutrient-packed foods, herbs, and spices, it goes a long way toward enhancing your health—and the health of everyone else in your household. Working toward long-term healthy eating habits, therefore, means taking a thorough inventory to decide which foods can stay and which should go. By purging unhealthy foods such as chips, frozen pizzas, soda, cookies, and sugary cereals, not only will you find it easier to follow a nutritious way of eating, but you'll also have more room for nutritious options.

Pantry

To get the ball rolling, let's take a look at the staples of healthy eating. There's no need to run out and buy every single item listed—instead, each week try to add a few foods you don't keep stocked. Having these inexpensive, ready-to-go basics for making meals will simplify your life while enhancing your household's health.

When you look into your cupboards or pantry, you should see foods that are high in fiber and protein and low in sugar, salt, and saturated fats. Following is a list of foods that meet the criteria:

Foods to Stock in the Pantry	
Canned or dried beans, lentils, and split peas	Popcorn
Canned refried beans, fat free	Potatoes and sweet potatoes
Canned broths, low sodium	Seeds such as chia, flax, hemp, pumpkin, and sunflower
Canned vegetables, low sodium or no salt added	Spaghetti sauce
Canned tomatoes, tomato sauce, and tomato paste, no salt added	Vinegars such as balsamic, red wine, and white wine
Canned fruits, unsweetened or packed in own juice	Whole grain cereals (at least 5 grams of fiber per serving)
Canned tuna, salmon, or chicken, water packed	Whole grains such as barley, buckwheat, bulgur, brown rice, and farro
Dried fruit	100 percent whole wheat bread (at least 2 grams of fiber per serving)
Healthy oils such as olive or canola and nonstick cooking spray	Whole wheat crackers (at least 2 grams of fiber per serving)
Nuts, including peanuts, unsalted	Whole wheat pasta
Nut butters such as natural peanut and almond butter	Whole wheat tortillas
Steel-cut, rolled, or quick-cooking oats (not instant)	Various spices such as cinnamon, paprika, and garlic powder; dried herbs such as thyme and basil

Here is a short list of foods to remove from your pantry. Many of these highly processed foods are sources of unhealthy saturated or trans fats, high levels of sodium, refined and low-fiber grains, and added sugars.

Foods to Remove from the Pantry	
Cake, brownie, and other dessert mixes	Sugary beverages such as soda, sports drinks, lemonade, and sweetened tea mixes
Candy, jams and jellies	Chips, cookies, crackers (not whole wheat), and pretzels
Granola bars	Sugary breakfast cereals (more than 6 grams of sugar per serving)

Refrigerator and Freezer

Modern-day appliances provide the luxury of eating a wide variety of nutritious foods year-round. Following are foods you should see when you open your refrigerator or freezer.

Foods to Stock in the Refrigerator and Freezer	
Eggs	Lean animal proteins such as beef, chicken, fish, pork, lamb, and turkey
Fresh fruit and vegetables	Leftovers or cooked extras, such as beans, rice, or quinoa
Fresh herbs	Low-fat cheese, including fresh mozzarella, cottage cheese, Parmesan, and string cheese
Frozen edamame	Mustard, Dijon
Frozen vegetables, without sauce	Nonfat or low-fat milk and nondairy plant-based alternatives such as almond or soy milk
Frozen fruits, unsweetened	Greek yogurt, nonfat or low-fat
Leafy greens such as arugula, kale, and spinach	Hummus

Foods to Remove from the Refrigerator and Freezer	
Alcoholic beverages, unless in moderation	Gourmet ice cream
Butter or margarine, stick form	Processed meats such as bologna, hot dogs, sausage, or cold cuts
Fish sticks	Soda and other sweetened beverages
Frozen burritos, chicken nuggets, fish sticks, dinners, fries, and pizza	Creamy salad dressings

Two-Week Menu Plan

Without a plan, even the most well-thought-out ideas can veer off course, especially when it comes to making wise food choices. That's why having a two-week menu plan will not only get you started on eating healthy but also hold you accountable for reaching healthy weight goals by functioning as a template. This menu plan is simply a guide to get ideas from; feel free to switch up meals according to your personal schedule. Most of the meals are easily put together without a lot of prep work. And if there are leftovers, just have them the following day to save time and money.

By following this guide, you will get a better sense of how and what to eat. Even better, menu planning will save you time and money by helping you avoid eating out after a long day. When everything is already planned for the week, you can shop and meal prep on weekends so all you have to do is quickly put it together at each meal. Let's get started.

Week One				
	Breakfast	**Lunch**	**Dinner**	**Snack**
Monday	Greek yogurt with berries and walnuts, two slices whole grain toast	Tuna tossed with brown rice and lemon juice, leafy green salad	Whole wheat spaghetti with meatballs, mixed veggies, strawberries	Tangerine slices or any fruit, popcorn
Tuesday	Chocolate Banana Smoothie (page 193)—add in one scoop chocolate or vanilla whey protein powder to boost protein	Vegetarian Pasta Primavera (page 214)— add in chickpeas to boost protein	Slow-Cooker Chicken, Quinoa, & White Bean Chili (page 203), roasted potatoes, asparagus	Unsalted almonds, cut-up fresh veggies with hummus

	Breakfast	Lunch	Dinner	Snack
Wednesday	Whole grain cereal with milk, fruit	Mixed greens salad with leftover chopped chicken and cut-up veggies	Build-your-own tacos, refried beans, fresh fruit	Sliced apples, almonds or walnuts
Thursday	Protein-spiked yogurt parfait*	Chickpea Spinach Pasta Salad (page 213), melon slices	Dr. David Samadi's Mediterranean Salmon (page 200), brown rice, broccoli	Bean dip with whole grain crackers
Friday	Veggie Scrambled Eggs with Cheese (page 198)	Turkey sandwich, cut-up fresh veggies like carrots and zucchini	Citrus-Marinated Beef Top Sirloin and Fruit Kabobs (page 201), grilled corn	Blackberries with Sweet Almond Cashew Cream (page 222)

* Stir half a scoop of vanilla whey protein powder into a cup of plain Greek yogurt. Top with ½ cup frozen mixed berries, 2 tbsp. sliced almonds, and 1 tsp. ground flaxseed.

Week Two				
	Breakfast	Lunch	Dinner	Snack
Monday	One cup low-fat cottage cheese with fruit and chia or flaxseeds	Mixed greens salad with other veggies, chopped nuts, and feta cheese	Store-bought rotisserie chicken, baked sweet potato, green beans	String cheese, grapes or apple slices
Tuesday	Overnight Oats (page 195)	Whole wheat tortilla wrap with leftover rotisserie chicken, hummus, sun-dried tomatoes, and greens, fruit	Easy Salmon/Tuna Cakes (page 210), brown rice, cooked carrots and zucchini	Cut-up fresh veggies with hummus or Greek yogurt dip
Wednesday	Protein-spiked yogurt parfait*	Tomato Veggie Split Pea Soup (page 218), two mozzarella cheese sticks	Sweet Potato Frittata (page 211), side salad, mixed berries	Black Bean and Corn Salsa (page 220) with whole wheat pita bread

Continued on next page

	Breakfast	Lunch	Dinner	Snack
Thursday	Brain-Boosting Berry Smoothie (page 194)—add in half scoop whey protein powder	Grilled cheese sandwich with tomato, mixed fruit	Baked fish, potatoes, steamed veggies	Hard-boiled egg with fruit
Friday	Spicy Breakfast Pizza (page 197)	Mixed greens salad with any leftover fish, nuts, other veggies, and fresh fruit	Beef Steak and Black Bean Soft Tacos (page 208), leafy green salad, watermelon	Tropical Mango Guacamole (page 221) with tortilla chips

* Stir half a scoop of vanilla whey protein powder into a cup of plain Greek yogurt. Top with ½ cup frozen mixed berries, 2 tbsp. sliced almonds, and 1 tsp. ground flaxseed.

BREAKFAST RECIPES

Chocolate Banana Smoothie

Top nutrients: Good source of protein and calcium; low sodium and low fat.

Why it's great for men: Making this smoothie with chocolate milk offers an easy, delicious option for exercise recovery. After a tough workout, chocolate milk has carbohydrates to refuel, protein to help repair and rebuild muscles, and fluids and electrolytes to help rehydrate and replenish critical nutrients lost in sweat. Low-fat chocolate milk also has the carb to protein ratio scientifically shown to refuel exhausted muscles quickly (https://builtwithchocolatemilk.com/).

Makes two 1-cup servings

Ingredients
1 teaspoon vanilla extract
1 very ripe banana, peeled, frozen
1 cup fat-free white milk or chocolate milk
1 teaspoon unsweetened cocoa powder (if made with white milk; optional)

Directions
1. Combine all ingredients in a blender.
2. Cover and blend until smooth. Serve immediately.

Nutrition: If using fat-free chocolate milk—140 calories; 0 grams total fat; 0 grams saturated fat; 3 milligrams cholesterol; 5 grams protein; 30 grams carbohydrates; 2 grams fiber; 91 milligrams sodium; 153 milligrams calcium. If using fat-free white milk—100 calories; 0 grams total fat; 0 grams saturated fat; 5 milligrams cholesterol; 5 grams protein; 20 grams carbohydrates; 2 grams fiber; 55 milligrams sodium; 154 milligrams calcium.

Recipe courtesy of www.milklife.com

Brain-Boosting Berry Smoothie

Top nutrients: Great source of vitamins A and C, omega-3 fatty acids, antioxidants, and fiber.

Why it's great for men: Research shows that powerful antioxidants and phytochemicals in berries may improve cognitive functioning and memory. What's good for the brain is good for other parts of our body too, so be sure to try this tasty, unforgettable, brain cell–supporting smoothie.

Makes two 1¼-cup servings

Ingredients
½ cup orange juice
1 cup plain Greek yogurt
1½ cups frozen blueberries
½ cup frozen raspberries
1–2 tablespoons chia seeds
¼ cup walnuts

Directions
1. Combine the orange juice and yogurt in a blender.
2. Add the blueberries, raspberries, chia seeds, and walnuts.
3. Blend until smooth.

Nutrition: 180 calories; 2 grams total fat; 0 grams saturated fat; 0 milligrams cholesterol; 10 grams protein; 30 grams carbohydrates; 5 grams fiber; 35 milligrams sodium.

Overnight Oats

Top nutrients: Excellent source of protein and calcium; low sodium. This recipe contains a healthy source of fat from the walnuts.

Why it's great for men: Overnight oats are easy to throw together ahead of time, and using milk instead of water adds high-quality protein and other nutrients such as calcium, potassium, and vitamin D.

Makes one serving

Ingredients
⅓ cup old-fashioned rolled oats (not quick-cooking or instant)
½ cup fat-free or low-fat milk
¼ teaspoon vanilla extract
2 tablespoons mixed fresh or dried fruit, chopped
1 tablespoon toasted walnuts, chopped
1 tablespoon honey
1 cup (8 ounces) fat-free or low-fat milk

Directions
1. Combine the oats, milk, and vanilla in a bowl or jar.
2. Cover and refrigerate overnight.
3. In the morning before serving, stir in the fresh or dried fruit, nuts, and honey.
4. Enjoy with a glass of milk.

Nutrition: 400 calories; 6 grams total fat; 0 grams saturated fat; 10 milligrams cholesterol; 18 grams protein; 68 grams carbohydrates; 4 grams fiber; 180 milligrams sodium; 470 milligrams calcium.

Recipe courtesy of www.milklife.com

Apricot and Tahini Steel Cut Oats with Cinnamon

Top nutrients: Good source of protein and fiber; low fat and low sodium.

Why it's great for men: If you want to boost fiber and fruit in a meal, try this recipe. It requires a little bit of extra cooking time than regular oatmeal but is well worth it. If tahini is unfamiliar to you, it's a store-bought paste made from sesame seeds that is commonly used in Mediterranean and Middle Eastern cooking.

Makes two servings

Ingredients
1½ cups milk
½ cup steel cut oats, uncooked
2 fresh apricots, diced, or add 4 chopped, dried apricots to each bowl
1 tablespoon tahini
1 teaspoon honey
Cinnamon, to taste

Directions
1. In a small pot, bring milk and oats to a boil, then add the apricots, tahini, and honey. Stir to combine.
2. Cover, reduce heat, and simmer for 15 to 20 minutes, stirring occasionally.
3. Remove from heat and let stand covered 5 minutes. Divide oatmeal into two bowls, then top each bowl with a sprinkle of cinnamon.

Nutrition: 290 calories; 7 grams total fat; 1 gram saturated fat; 0 milligrams cholesterol; 13 grams protein; 45 grams carbohydrates; 5 grams fiber; 80 grams sodium.

Recipe courtesy of Oldways Whole Grains Council, www.wholegrainscouncil.org

Spicy Breakfast Pizza

Top nutrients: Excellent source of protein and calcium; low sodium.

Why it's great for men: Who doesn't love a good pizza? This recipe is simple to make and is ready in less than thirty minutes. It's also an easy way to get a variety of nutritious foods, including milk, olive oil, eggs, asparagus, arugula, and whole grains.

Makes six servings

Ingredients

4 eggs

2 tablespoons fat-free or low-fat milk

1 teaspoon olive oil

1 cup fresh asparagus, cut into
  1-inch pieces

1 tablespoon fresh chives or green
  onions, minced

1 12-inch prepared whole wheat
  pizza crust

¾ cup shredded part-skim
  mozzarella cheese

1 cup fresh arugula

Sriracha sauce (optional)

Directions

1. Preheat oven to 425 degrees F.

2. Whisk the eggs and milk together in a small bowl.

3. Coat a large nonstick skillet with cooking spray. Heat the pan over medium heat. Add the olive oil. Add the asparagus and cook 3 to 5 minutes or until slightly softened.

4. Stir in the egg mixture and cook just until set, stirring frequently with a rubber spatula. Do not overcook. Remove skillet from the heat and fold in the chives.

5. To assemble the pizza, spoon the egg mixture onto the pizza crust. Sprinkle with mozzarella cheese and bake until cheese is melted, about 5 minutes.

6. Top with arugula and drizzle with Sriracha sauce to taste. Cut into six wedges and serve with an 8-ounce glass of milk.

Nutrition: 210 calories; 7 grams total fat; 3 grams saturated fat; 135 milligrams cholesterol; 18 grams protein; 18 grams carbohydrates; 1 gram fiber; 280 milligrams sodium.

Recipe courtesy of www.milklife.com

Veggie Scrambled Eggs with Cheese

Top nutrients: Source of protein, vitamins A and C, antioxidants, and fiber.

Why it's great for men: Looking for something different besides cold cereal or toast? This breakfast has it all—lots of protein, veggies, and additional nutrients when you add a side of fruit. Getting in veggies early in the day can be tough, but this recipe makes it super easy.

Makes two 1-cup servings

Ingredients

1 tablespoon olive oil

5 eggs

Salt and pepper, to taste

2 cups washed baby spinach, chopped

3 green onions, thinly sliced, both green and white parts

12 cherry tomatoes, halved or quartered

2 tablespoons fresh basil, chopped

½ cup shredded cheese of your choice, plus additional for garnishing

Directions

1. Heat skillet over medium-high heat and add olive oil.
2. Whisk eggs together in a bowl, and season with salt and pepper.
3. Add spinach and green onions to the preheated skillet. Sauté until spinach is slightly wilted, less than 1 minute.
4. Add egg mixture to the pan and stir constantly with a spatula. When eggs are almost set, add cherry tomatoes, basil, and cheese. Continue to stir constantly to mix ingredients.
5. When eggs are set, remove from pan, garnish with shredded cheese, and serve immediately.

Nutrition: 138 calories; 10 grams total fat; 4 grams saturated fat; 280 milligrams cholesterol; 10 grams protein; 2 grams carbohydrates; 2 grams fiber; 85 milligrams sodium.

Banana Muffins

Top nutrients: Low fat; good source of fiber, protein, and some omega-3 fatty acids.

Why it's great for men: Never discard an overripe banana again—reduce food waste while upping the nutritional value of this favorite baked good. This tasty whole wheat recipe comes together in no time using common foods in your kitchen. Refuel with these muffins post workout to restore muscle glycogen from healthy carbs and a good dose of quality protein.

Makes ten muffins

Ingredients

3 overripe bananas

2 large eggs

2 cups whole wheat pastry flour (or white whole wheat flour)

⅓ cup sugar

1 teaspoon salt

1 teaspoon baking soda

½ cup walnuts, chopped

Directions

1. Preheat oven to 350 degrees F. Lightly grease and flour 10 cups of a muffin tin.
2. Mix bananas and eggs together thoroughly with an electric mixer.
3. Sift dry ingredients (flour, sugar, salt, baking soda) together. Add to bananas and eggs.
4. Add nuts while mixing just until everything is combined. (Overmixing makes muffins dense.)
5. Spoon into muffin tins, filling each cup about ¾ full.
6. Bake for 20 minutes or until a toothpick comes out clean.

Note: You can stretch this to a dozen muffins, but they'll be smaller. If you use a 9x5 loaf pan instead, increase baking time to about one hour, then test with a toothpick.

Nutrition: 200 calories per muffin; 5 grams total fat; 0.5 grams saturated fat; 50 milligrams cholesterol; 5 grams protein; 34 grams carbohydrates; 5 grams fiber; 370 milligrams sodium.

Recipe courtesy of Oldways Whole Grains Council, www.wholegrainscouncil.org

LUNCH AND DINNER RECIPES

Dr. David Samadi's Mediterranean Salmon

Top nutrients: Excellent source of protein, vitamin B12, omega-3 fatty acids, potassium, and selenium.

Why it's great for men: If you're intimidated to cook fish, here is a fearless recipe that makes it easy. In twenty minutes, you can be eating a flavor-filled salmon, rich in brain- and heart-boosting monounsaturated fat and omega-3 fatty acids. Having two fish meals a week may lower the risk for heart attack, stroke, and cognitive decline.

Makes four 3-ounce fillets

Ingredients

½ cup olive oil

¼ cup balsamic vinegar

4 cloves garlic, pressed

4 3-ounce fillets

1 tablespoon fresh cilantro, chopped

1 tablespoon fresh basil, chopped

1½ teaspoons garlic salt

Directions

1. Mix together olive oil and balsamic vinegar in a small bowl.
2. Arrange salmon fillets in a shallow baking dish. Rub pressed garlic onto the fillets, then pour the vinegar and oil over them, turning once to coat.
3. Season with cilantro, basil, and garlic salt. Set aside to marinate for 10 minutes.
4. Preheat oven's broiler. Place the dish about 6 inches from the heat source and broil for 15 minutes, brushing occasionally with the sauce from the dish and turning once or until browned on both sides and easily flaked with a fork.

Nutrition: 235 calories; 12 grams total fat; 4 grams saturated fat; 60 milligrams cholesterol; 30 grams protein; 2 grams carbohydrates; 1 gram fiber; 50 milligrams sodium.

Recipe courtesy of Dr. David Samadi, Urologic Oncologist Expert and Renowned Robotic Surgeon, www.prostatecancer911.com

Citrus-Marinated Beef Top Sirloin and Fruit Kabobs

Top nutrients: Excellent source of protein, vitamin B12, iron, and zinc.

Why it's great for men: Made with lean beef, this recipe is good eating with a twist. Low in total and saturated fat, rich in iron and zinc, and full of antioxidants from the fruit, your health—and taste buds—have it made with this mouthwatering meal.

Makes four servings—1 skewer steak and 1 skewer fruit

Ingredients

1 medium orange

¼ cup fresh cilantro, chopped

1 tablespoon smoked paprika

¼ teaspoon ground red pepper (optional)

1 beef top sirloin steak center cut, boneless (about 1 pound)

4 cups mango, watermelon, peaches, and/or plums, cubed

Additional cilantro for garnishing (optional)

Directions

1. Grate orange peel and squeeze 2 tablespoons juice from orange; reserve juice.
2. Combine orange peel, cilantro, paprika, and red pepper, if desired, in small bowl.
3. Cut beef steak into 1¼–inch pieces.
4. Place beef and 2½ tablespoons cilantro mixture in food-safe plastic bag; turn to coat.
5. Place remaining cilantro mixture and fruit in separate food-safe plastic bag; turn to coat.
6. Close bags securely. Marinate beef and fruit in refrigerator 15 minutes to 2 hours.
7. Soak eight 9-inch bamboo skewers in water for 10 minutes. Thread beef evenly onto four skewers, leaving a small space between pieces. Thread fruit onto four remaining skewers.

8. Place kabobs on grill over medium, ash-covered coals. Grill beef kabobs covered, 5 to 7 minutes (over medium heat on preheated gas grill for 7 to 8 minutes) for medium rare (145 degrees F) to medium (160 degrees F) doneness, turning occasionally. Grill fruit kabobs 5 to 7 minutes or until softened and beginning to brown, turning once.
9. Drizzle reserved orange juice over fruit kabobs. Garnish with cilantro, if desired.

Nutrition: 239 calories; 5.7 grams total fat; 1.8 grams saturated fat; 69 milligrams cholesterol; 28 grams protein; 22 grams carbohydrates; 3.4 grams fiber; 53 milligrams sodium.

Recipe courtesy of www.beefitswhatsfordinner.com

Slow-Cooker Chicken, Quinoa, & White Bean Chili

Top nutrients: Excellent source of protein; good source of calcium.

Why it's great for men: You can throw nearly everything into a slow cooker and come home a few hours later to an almost-ready meal. All you have to do is add the beans, shred the chicken, and add toppings. It's also an easy way to incorporate nutritious but unfamiliar foods like quinoa.

Makes nine 1-cup servings

Ingredients
1 pound uncooked boneless, skinless chicken breast
¾ cup uncooked quinoa
2 cups low-sodium chicken broth
1½ cups milk
3 cups (24 ounces) mild jarred salsa verde (or mild salsa of choice)
2 cloves garlic, minced
1 medium yellow onion, diced
2 bell peppers, diced
2 cups frozen corn
1 tablespoon cumin
30 ounces canned white beans (cannellini, great northern, etc.),
    drained and rinsed
Fresh cilantro, chopped (optional)
Green onions, sliced (optional)
Shredded cheese (optional)
Sour cream (optional)
Avocado, cubed (optional)
Tortilla chips (optional)

Directions

1. Combine all ingredients except beans in slow cooker and stir well to combine.
2. Cover and cook for 2½ to 3 hours on high or 5 to 6 hours on low, until chicken breast is fully cooked and can be pulled apart easily with two forks.
3. Stir in beans. Transfer chicken breast from slow cooker to a plate or cutting board and, using two forks, shred well. Return shredded chicken to the slow cooker and stir well to incorporate.
4. Spoon into bowl and top with cilantro, sliced green onions, shredded cheese, sour cream, and avocado. Serve with tortilla chips, if desired.

Nutrition: 320 calories; 4 grams total fat; 0.5 grams saturated fat; 30 milligrams cholesterol; 23 grams protein; 47 grams carbohydrates; 9 grams fiber; 530 milligrams sodium.

Recipe courtesy of www.milklife.com

Top Sirloin Steak and Green Bean & Tomato Salad

Top nutrients: Excellent source of protein, iron, and zinc.

Why it's great for men: This fresh, colorful meal, certified by the American Heart Association as a heart-healthy recipe, is perfect for boosting your intake of muscle-building protein and is a good dose of zinc—45 percent of the daily value. Zinc plays an important role in producing testosterone. Many adults do not get enough zinc, and if you are deficient in this mineral, it may lead to erectile dysfunction.

Makes four servings

Ingredients

1 pound beef top sirloin steak, boneless, cut ¾-inch thick
¼ cup plus 2 tablespoons reduced-fat balsamic vinaigrette, divided
2½ cups fresh green beans, cut into 2-inch pieces
1 teaspoon olive oil
1 cup tomatoes, cut in half
Salt and pepper, to taste
5 cups fresh baby spinach (about one 5-ounce package)
¼ cup shaved Parmesan cheese

Directions

1. Cut beef steak lengthwise in half, then crosswise into ⅛-to-¼-inch-thick strips. Combine 2 tablespoons vinaigrette dressing and beef in medium bowl; toss to coat. Cover and marinate in refrigerator 30 minutes to 2 hours.
2. Heat large nonstick skillet over medium-high heat until hot. Add green beans and olive oil; stir-fry 5 minutes. Add tomatoes; stir-fry 2 to 3 minutes or until beans are crisp-tender and tomatoes begin to brown slightly. Remove from skillet; salt and pepper as desired. Keep warm.
3. Add to same skillet half of beef; stir-fry 1 to 3 minutes or until outside surface of beef is no longer pink. Remove from skillet. Repeat with remaining steak.
4. Divide spinach evenly among four plates. Top with beef and vegetables. Sprinkle with cheese. Drizzle with remaining ¼ cup dressing.

Nutrition: 230 calories; 9 grams total fat; 2.9 grams saturated fat; 72 milligrams cholesterol; 30 grams protein; 12 grams carbohydrates; 3.2 grams fiber; 448 milligrams sodium.

Recipe courtesy of www.beefitswhatsfordinner.com

Easy Walnut-Crusted Salmon

Top nutrients: Excellent source of protein, potassium, and heart-healthy mono-unsaturated fat and omega-3 fatty acids.

Why it's great for men: This top-notch recipe uses heart-healthy salmon and walnuts combined with delicately flavored hints of honey and mustard for a quick and easy meal. Pair it with a spinach salad loaded with cut-up veggies for a perfect dinner.

Makes four salmon fillet servings

Ingredients

4 4-ounce boneless salmon fillets

¼ teaspoon salt

¼ teaspoon black pepper

½ cup whole wheat breadcrumbs

1 cup walnuts

1 clove garlic, minced

1 tablespoon honey

1 tablespoon Dijon mustard

4 teaspoons olive oil

Directions

1. Preheat oven to 425 degrees F and line a rimmed baking sheet with parchment paper.
2. Sprinkle both sides of the salmon fillets with salt and pepper. Set aside.
3. Pulse breadcrumbs, walnuts, garlic, honey, and mustard in a food processor until well combined. Place mixture in a shallow dish.
4. Press salmon fillets into mixture to coat on all sides. Place fillets on the prepared baking sheet and drizzle with olive oil.
5. Bake the fillets for 10 to 12 minutes until golden brown on top and cooked all the way through.

Note: Four 4-ounce chicken tenders can be substituted for the salmon fillets. Reduce oven temperature to 350 degrees F and bake for about 45 minutes.

Nutrition: 230 calories; 12 grams total fat; 2 grams saturated fat; 65 milligrams cholesterol; 24 grams protein; 4 grams carbohydrates; 1 gram fiber; 250 milligrams sodium.

Beef Steak and Black Bean Soft Tacos

Top nutrients: Excellent source of fiber, protein, iron, niacin, thiamine, vitamin B6, vitamin B12, zinc, and selenium; good source of choline.

Why it's great for men: This heart-healthy recipe, certified by the American Heart Association, makes a mouthwatering meal with an extra flavor boost from black beans, salsa, and fresh toppings. You'll enjoy its robust taste while feeding your body with healthy nutrients.

Makes four servings

Ingredients
1 cup salsa, divided
2 teaspoons chili powder
1½ teaspoons ground cumin, divided
1 pound beef bottom round steaks, cut ¼-inch thick
1 15-ounce can no-salt-added black beans
8 small corn tortillas (5-to-6-inch diameter), warmed
1 cup tomatoes, diced
½ cup lettuce, shredded
½ cup red onion, diced
2 tablespoons plus 2 teaspoons fresh cilantro, chopped
1 medium ripe avocado, cut into 8 thin slices
1 lime, cut into 8 wedges

Directions
1. Combine ½ cup salsa, chili powder, and 1 teaspoon cumin. Place beef steaks in food-safe plastic bag; turn to coat. Close bag securely and marinate in refrigerator 6 hours or as long as overnight, turning occasionally.
2. Combine 1 cup black beans, remaining ½ cup salsa, and remaining ½ teaspoon cumin in medium microwave-safe bowl. Mash with fork into chunky paste. Cover and microwave on high 1 to 2 minutes or until hot, stirring once. Keep warm.

3. Meanwhile, heat large nonstick skillet over medium-high heat until hot; remove from heat and coat with nonstick spray. Remove steaks from marinade; discard marinade. Cooking batches, if necessary, place steaks in skillet (do not overcrowd) and cook 2 to 3 minutes for medium rare (145 degrees F) doneness, turning once. Do not overcook. Remove steaks from skillet; keep warm. Repeat with remaining steaks.

4. Spread bean mixture evenly on tortillas. Cut steaks into 4 pieces each and divide evenly among tortillas. Top beans with remaining ½ cup beans, tomatoes, lettuce, red onion, cilantro, avocado, and lime wedges, as desired. Fold tortillas in half to serve.

Note: Steaks may be cut into bite-sized pieces in step 4.

Nutrition: 478 calories; 16 grams total fat; 3 grams saturated fat; 66 milligrams cholesterol; 36 grams protein; 56 grams carbohydrates; 13.6 grams fiber; 450 milligrams sodium.

Recipe courtesy of www.beefitswhatsfordinner.com

Easy Salmon/Tuna Cakes

Top nutrients: Excellent source of protein, omega-3 fatty acids, selenium, potassium, and vitamins A and C; low carbohydrate and low fat.

Why it's great for men: Looking for a simple, quick, inexpensive, and healthy meal that takes less than ten minutes to make? This tasty recipe is chock-full of nutrients promoting both brain and heart health. Use either salmon or tuna, whichever you prefer.

Makes four 3-ounce servings

Ingredients

2 6-ounce cans or pouches of salmon or tuna

2 eggs, beaten

½ cup onion, finely chopped

½ cup bell peppers, green or red, finely diced

½ teaspoon salt

½ teaspoon pepper

2 teaspoons lemon juice

6–8 tablespoons finely ground breadcrumbs (bought or homemade)

4 teaspoons olive oil

Directions

1. Mix salmon or tuna with beaten egg, onions, and bell peppers.
2. Season with salt, pepper, and lemon juice; stir together.
3. Mix in 2 tablespoons breadcrumbs.
4. Form into palm-sized patties and coat with additional breadcrumbs.
5. Heat olive oil in a pan or skillet over medium-high heat.
6. Place patties in oil, cooking about 2 to 3 minutes to brown before turning over once to cook the other side until browned.

Note: This recipe can be prepped the night before—after step 4, place formed patties on a plate, cover with plastic wrap, and refrigerate until ready to cook in step 5.

Nutrition: 180 calories; 10 grams total fat; 2 grams saturated fat; 25 milligrams cholesterol; 20 grams protein; 2 grams carbohydrates; 1 gram fiber; 315 milligrams sodium.

Sweet Potato Frittata

Top nutrients: Excellent source of calcium and protein; good source of fiber and antioxidants; low carbohydrate.

Why it's great for men: Here's an easy recipe packed with healthy ingredients, making it a standout among other egg dishes. Frittatas are an Italian dish perfect for showing off creativity and getting in extra veggies men may bypass. Feel free to add in other vegetables such as sliced mushrooms, bite-sized pieces of asparagus, broccoli, zucchini, tomatoes, or even eggplant to ramp up its nutritional power.

Makes six servings

Ingredients
2 tablespoons olive oil
¼ cup red onion, finely chopped
1 red bell pepper, diced
1 medium sweet potato, peeled, cut into bite-sized chunks
2 cups baby kale
6 eggs
¼ cup low-fat milk
½ teaspoon salt
¼ teaspoon pepper
½ teaspoon thyme
½ cup shredded mozzarella cheese

Directions
1. Preheat oven to 375 degrees F. Coat a 10-inch oven-safe skillet with nonstick cooking spray.
2. Add olive oil to the skillet and heat over medium-high heat on stovetop.
3. Add red onion, bell pepper, and sweet potato to olive oil. Sauté in hot oil until soft, 6 to 8 minutes.
4. Add kale to skillet and stir to wilt.
5. Vigorously whisk eggs with ¼ cup milk, salt, pepper, and thyme in a separate bowl.

6. Pour egg mixture over vegetables in the skillet; cook for 4 to 5 minutes or until edges begin to set.
7. Sprinkle with mozzarella cheese.
8. Transfer skillet to preheated oven for an additional 10 to 14 minutes or until slightly puffed and set.

Nutrition: 200 calories; 13 grams total fat; 4 grams saturated fat; 248 milligrams cholesterol; 12 grams protein; 10 grams carbohydrates; 2 grams fiber; 368 milligrams sodium.

SOUPS, SIDES, AND SALAD RECIPES

Chickpea Spinach Pasta Salad

Top nutrients: Great source of fiber and protein.

Why it's great for men: This is a perfect recipe to make on a weekend for a busy week ahead. Served chilled or at room temperature, this flavorful, simple, and economical meal is ready in no time.

Makes four servings

Ingredients

6 ounces uncooked whole wheat (or other whole grain) pasta— rotini recommended

Juice of one lemon

3 tablespoons extra-virgin olive oil

2 cloves garlic, minced

4 cups fresh spinach leaves, chopped

1 15-ounce can chickpeas (garbanzo beans), drained and rinsed

2 ounces crumbled feta cheese

Directions

1. Bring a large pot of water to a boil and cook pasta according to package directions (about 8 minutes, usually).
2. While pasta is cooking, mix lemon juice, olive oil, and garlic in a very large salad bowl.
3. When pasta is done, drain and put in the bowl so it can absorb the lemon sauce.
4. Add chickpeas and spinach and toss thoroughly. Sprinkle with feta cheese when ready to serve.

Nutrition: 411 calories; 15 grams total fat; 4 grams saturated fat; 0 milligrams cholesterol; 14 grams protein; 59 grams carbohydrates; 5 grams fiber; 498 milligrams sodium.

Recipe courtesy of Oldways Whole Grains Council, www.wholegrainscouncil.org

Vegetarian Pasta Primavera

Top nutrients: Excellent source of fiber, vitamins A, C, E, and K, folate, magnesium, beta-carotene, and lutein; good source of protein; low fat and low sodium.

Why it's great for men: If you're looking to include more veggies in a meal, this recipe fulfills that need. Whole wheat pasta makes a perfect base for the veggies, increasing fiber, phosphorus, magnesium, and folate. It's a delicious and nutritious meal as is or with cut-up cooked chicken or beef added for a protein and iron boost.

Makes four servings (½ cup pasta and ½ cup vegetables)

Ingredients
8 ounces whole wheat pasta—spaghetti, rotini, bowtie, or your choice
1 cup each of broccoli, cauliflower, and carrots, cut into bite-sized pieces
1 cup frozen peas
2–4 teaspoons olive oil
2 teaspoons red wine vinegar
2 teaspoons lemon juice
1 cup tomato, cut into chunks
1–2 tablespoons fresh basil, chopped
Parmesan cheese, if desired

Directions
1. Follow directions for cooking pasta.
2. Meanwhile, bring a large saucepan of salted water to a boil; add in broccoli, cauliflower, and carrots and frozen peas. Cook for about 3 to 5 minutes or until crisp-tender.
3. While vegetables and pasta are cooking, prepare olive oil dressing by mixing the oil, vinegar, and lemon juice.
4. Drain pasta and vegetables into separate colanders.

5. Place pasta on a plate, spoon cooked vegetables over the pasta, then add in chunks of tomato and chopped fresh basil.
6. Drizzle pasta and vegetables with olive oil dressing. If desired, sprinkle with Parmesan cheese.

Note: If desired, add in a protein such as cooked beef or chicken in step 5.

Nutrition (without an added protein source): 252 calories; 4.5 grams total fat; 0 grams saturated fat; 0 grams cholesterol; 8 grams protein; 45 grams carbohydrates; 12 grams fiber; 75 milligrams sodium.

Lemon Broccoli with Dried Cherries

Top nutrients: Source of vitamins A, C, and K, omega-3 fatty acids, fiber, folate, magnesium, beta-carotene, and lutein.

Why it's great for men: Who says men don't like green food? If you're not a fan, you will be after this recipe. From the tangy dressing to the hint of sweetness from the cherries to the health-enhancing broccoli loaded with valuable nutrients, you won't want to pass this up.

Makes four ½-cup servings

Ingredients

1 large head of broccoli, cut into florets, stems peeled and sliced ½ inch
¼ cup extra-virgin olive oil
2 tablespoons red wine vinegar
½ tablespoon fresh lemon juice
1 teaspoon lemon zest, finely grated
½ small shallot, minced
½ cup dried cherries
Kosher salt and black pepper, to taste

Directions

1. Fill a large saucepan with salted water and bring to a boil.
2. Add broccoli florets and cook for about 5 minutes or until bright green and tender. Drain into a colander and rinse immediately with cold water to stop the cooking; pat dry.
3. In a large bowl, whisk olive oil with the red wine vinegar, lemon juice, lemon zest, shallot, and dried cherries. Season with salt and pepper.
4. Add the broccoli, toss to coat, and serve.

Nutrition: 162 calories; 6 grams total fat; 0.5 grams saturated fat; 0 milligrams cholesterol; 2 grams protein; 25 grams carbohydrates; 6 grams fiber; 50 milligrams sodium.

Creamy Key Lime Fruit Salad

Top nutrients: Source of vitamins A, C, E, and K, fiber, antioxidants, beta-carotene, lutein, and zeaxanthin.

Why it's great for men: This is a tried-and-true fruit salad without the excessive sugar or fat other fruit salads often rely on. This one uses yogurt to give it a hint of sweetness while bringing out the tantalizing mix of fruit flavors. An enticing dessert, breakfast, or snack, it also provides a nice blend of important antioxidants and fiber.

Makes eight ½-cup servings

Ingredients
¼ cup flaked or shredded coconut, toasted
2 6-ounce containers key lime pie–flavored Greek yogurt
4 tablespoons freshly squeezed orange juice
2 cups fresh pineapple chunks
1 cup strawberries, halved
2 cups green grapes, halved or whole
1 cup blueberries
2 cups cantaloupe, cubed

Directions
1. To toast coconut, heat a skillet over medium-low heat. Add coconut, stirring frequently for 6 to 12 minutes until golden brown.
2. Mix yogurt and orange juice in a bowl.
3. Layer fruit in order listed in the ingredients in a large clear glass bowl.
4. Pour yogurt mixture over fruit and sprinkle with toasted coconut. Serve immediately.

Note: If preferred, replace key lime pie–flavored Greek yogurt with vanilla Greek yogurt and call the recipe Creamy Vanilla Fruit Salad instead.

Nutrition: 130 calories; 2 grams total fat; 1 gram saturated fat; 0 milligrams cholesterol; 10 grams protein; 26 grams carbohydrates; 3 grams fiber; 15 grams sodium.

Tomato Veggie Split Pea Soup

Top nutrients: Excellent source of fiber, vitamins A, C, E, and K, antioxidants, and potassium; good source of protein; low fat.

Why it's great for men: Every hearty, wholesome spoonful of this soup is loaded with antioxidant-rich veggies you may be lacking in your diet. Besides tremendous amounts of fiber and health-enhancing nutrients, soups are generally good for hydration and creating a full feeling. Pair this with crusty bread, and you have a meal made in heaven.

Makes eight ½-cup servings

Ingredients

1 tablespoon extra-virgin olive oil
½ large onion, finely chopped
1 stalk celery, diced
2 cloves garlic, finely minced
2 large carrots, chopped into
  bite-sized pieces
1 cup frozen corn
1 14.5-ounce can black beans,
  drained and rinsed

½ medium zucchini, chopped into
  bite-sized pieces
2 cubes low-sodium chicken bouillon
1 teaspoon thyme
¼ teaspoon black pepper
2 14.5-ounce cans petite tomatoes,
  undrained
1 cup dried green split peas
  or dried lentils
4 cups water

Directions

1. Heat oil in 3-quart saucepan over medium heat. Cook onion, celery, and garlic in oil about 5 minutes or until softened.
2. Stir in remaining ingredients. Turn up heat to boiling, and then reduce heat to a simmer. Cover and simmer about 20 to 30 minutes or until heated through.

Nutrition: 190 calories; 2 grams total fat; 1 gram saturated fat; 0 milligrams cholesterol; 13 grams protein; 30 grams carbohydrates; 12 grams fiber; 150 milligrams sodium.

Oven-Roasted Lemon Parmesan Asparagus

Top nutrients: Good source of fiber, folate, and healthy monounsaturated fat and omega-3 fatty acids.

Why it's great for men: While you may steer clear of strong-flavored veggies like asparagus, roasting helps to caramelize the flavor, significantly reducing the natural bitterness. Asparagus provides a good source of nutrients such as vitamins A and C, helping boost men's immune functioning.

Makes four 1-cup servings

Ingredients

1 bunch of asparagus spears
3 tablespoons extra-virgin olive oil
1 tablespoon Parmesan cheese
1 clove garlic, chopped
1 teaspoon salt
½ teaspoon pepper
1 tablespoon fresh lemon juice

Directions

1. Preheat oven to 425 degrees F.
2. Wash and trim asparagus.
3. Place asparagus in a single layer on a baking sheet. Drizzle olive oil over spears, then toss spears to coat.
4. Evenly sprinkle Parmesan cheese, garlic, salt, and pepper over spears, then drizzle spears with lemon juice.
5. Bake until tender, about 12 to 15 minutes.

Nutrition: 113 calories; 5 grams total fat; 0.5 grams saturated fat; 0 milligrams cholesterol; 2 grams protein; 12 grams carbohydrates; 3 grams fiber; 45 milligrams sodium.

Black Bean and Corn Salsa

Top nutrients: Good source of fiber, protein, antioxidants, vitamin C, and lutein.

Why it's great for men: This is the perfect salsa to enjoy while watching the big game or out with the family on a picnic. Paired with chips or pita bread or even served over grilled meat, this salsa will get rave reviews. Not only does it taste great, but it's loaded with health benefits and takes just five minutes to make.

Makes eight ½-cup servings

Ingredients

1 15-ounce can low-sodium black beans, drained and rinsed
1 11-ounce can low-sodium whole kernel corn, drained
1 14.5-ounce can low-sodium petite diced tomatoes, drained
½ cup green onions, chopped
2 tablespoons fresh cilantro, chopped
½ cup Italian salad dressing
2 serrano chilies, seeded, chopped (optional)

Directions

1. Combine all ingredients together in a large bowl, mixing well.
2. Refrigerate until serving.

Nutrition: 144 calories; 8 grams total fat; 2 grams saturated fat; 0 milligrams cholesterol; 4 grams protein; 14 grams carbohydrates; 4 grams fiber; 90 milligrams sodium.

Tropical Mango Guacamole

Top nutrients: Excellent source of healthy monounsaturated fat and fiber; low sodium; good source of vitamins A, C, and E.

Why it's great for men: Here's a guac recipe you will come back for again and again. With the dazzling array of colors, great taste, ease of assembly, and key nutrients men require, this guac's a winner. It's a spin on a classic guacamole recipe thanks to a few unusual ingredients—mango, jicama, and pomegranate seeds. Trust me, you'll love it.

Makes eight ½-cup servings

Ingredients

1 ripe mango, diced into
   ¼-inch cubes
¼ cup jicama, diced into
   ¼-inch cubes
¼ cup red onion, finely chopped
¼ cup garlic, finely chopped
2 tablespoons fresh lemon juice

½ teaspoon salt
¼ teaspoon black pepper
2 ripe avocados, peeled, pits removed
2 tablespoons fresh cilantro, chopped
1 tablespoon red pomegranate seeds
   for garnishing (optional)

Directions

1. In a medium bowl, mix the mango, jicama, onion, garlic, lemon juice, salt, and pepper. Set aside.
2. In another bowl, add the avocado and mash until soft.
3. Add the mango mixture to the avocado and mix.
4. Top with cilantro and pomegranate seeds.

Nutrition: 251 calories; 15 grams total fat; 2 grams saturated fat; 0 milligrams cholesterol; 3 grams protein; 26 grams carbohydrates; 9 grams fiber; 300 milligrams sodium.

Recipe courtesy of the National Mango Board

Blackberries with Sweet Almond Cashew Cream

Top nutrients: Good source of fiber, manganese, monounsaturated fat, and antioxidants.

Why it's great for men: This sweet cream concoction not only pairs well with all types of berries (like blueberries, strawberries, and raspberries) but also offers less sugar and a healthier source of fat from cashews than dairy whipped cream. Besides its amazing taste, this recipe is antioxidant rich and good for heart, prostate, and brain health.

Makes four ½-cup servings

Ingredients
1 cup cashews
3 tablespoons maple syrup
¼ to ½ cup unsweetened vanilla almond milk
2 tablespoons lemon juice
Pinch of salt
½ teaspoon vanilla extract
Blackberries or other fresh berry of your choice

Directions
1. Place cashews in a medium bowl, cover with hot water, and soak for 30 minutes.
2. Drain cashews. Add cashews to a food processor along with the rest of the ingredients except berries. Blend together until smooth.
3. Serve with berries. Store cream in a covered container in the refrigerator up to 3 to 4 days.

Nutrition: 170 calories; 6 grams total fat; 1 gram saturated fat; 0 milligrams cholesterol; 3 grams protein; 26 grams carbohydrates; 4 grams fiber; 20 milligrams sodium.

REFERENCES

Introduction

1. Xu J, Murphy SL, Kochanek KD, Arias E. Mortality in the United States, 2018. NCHS Data Brief, no 355. National Center for Health Statistics. Reviewed January 2020. https://www.cdc.gov/nchs/products/databriefs/db355.htm

2. Wang H, Dwyer-Lindgren L, Lofgren KT, Rajaratnam JK, Marcus JR, Levin-Rector A, et al. Age-specific and sex-specific mortality in 187 countries, 1970-2010: a systematic analysis for the Global Burdens of Disease Study 2010. *Lancet.* 2012;380:2071–2094.

3. Thompson AE, Anisimowicz Y, Miedema B, Wodchis WP, Aubrey-Bassler K. The influence of gender and other patient characteristics on health care-seeking behaviour: a QUALICOPC study. *BMC Family Practice.* 2016;17:38.

4. Shmerling RH. Why men often die earlier than women. *Harvard Health Publishing* blog. Posted February 19, 2016. https://www.health.harvard.edu/blog/why-men-often-die-earlier-than-women-201602199137

Chapter 1

1. Rappleye, E. Women make 80 percent of healthcare decisions. Becker's Hospital Review. Updated 2015. https://www.beckershospitalreview.com/hospital-management-administration/women-make-80-percent-of-healthcare-decisions.html

2. Karlberg J, Chong DS, Lai WY. Do men have a higher case fatality rate of severe acute respiratory syndrome than women do? *Am J Epidemiol.* 2004;159(3):229–231.

3. Karlberg J, Chong DS, Lai WY. Do men have a higher case fatality rate of severe acute respiratory syndrome than women do? *Am J Epidemiol.* 2004;159(3):229–231.

4. Centers for Disease Control and Prevention. Current cigarette smoking among adults in the United States. Updated November 2019. https://www.cdc.gov/tobacco/data_statistics/fact_sheets/adult_data/cig_smoking/index.htm

5. Himmelstein MS, Sanchez DT. Masculinity impediments: internalized masculinity contributes to healthcare avoidance in men and women. *J Health Psychol.* 2016;21(7): 1283–1292.

6. Ramos E, Inés Zamudio M. In Chicago, 70% of Covid-19 deaths are black. WBEZ. Updated April 2020. https://www.wbez.org/stories/in-chicago-70-of-covid-19-deaths-are-black/dd3f295f-445e-4e38-b37f-a1503782b507

7. Macedo AC, Oliveira A, de Faria V. Boosting the immune system, from science to myth: analysis the infosphere with Google. *Front Med.* 2019;6:165.

Chapter 2

1. Miller AE, MacDougall JD, Tarnopolsky MA, Sale DG. Gender differences in strength and muscle fiber characteristics. *Eur J Appl Physiol Occup Physiol.* 1993;66(3):254–262.

2. National Institutes of Health. Sudden infant death syndrome (SIDS). U.S. Department of Health and Human Services. 2017. Accessed May 20, 2020. https://www.nichd.nih.gov /sites/default/files/publications/pubs/Documents/SIDS_QA_HealthCareProviders.pdf

3. Xu JQ, Murphy SL, Kochanek KD, Bastian BA. Deaths: final data for 2013. *Natl Vital Stat Rep.* 2016;64(2).

4. The Heart Foundation. Heart disease: scope and impact. Accessed May 20, 2020. https://theheartfoundation.org/heart-disease-facts-2/

5. American Cancer Society. Key statistics for lung cancer. 2019. Accessed May 20, 2020. https://www.cancer.org/cancer/lung-cancer/about/key-statistics.html

6. Barzi A, Pennell NA. Targeting angiogenesis in non-small cell lung cancer: agents in practice and clinical development. *European J Clin Med Oncol.* 2010 [cited 2016 Nov 21];2(1):31–42.

7. World Health Organization. *World Cancer Report 2008.* The International Agency for Research on Cancer; 2008. http://www.iarc.fr/en/publications/pdfs-online/wcr/2008 /wcr_2008.pdf

8. National Cancer Institute. Radon and cancer. 2011.

9. National Cancer Institute, Surveillance, Epidemiology, and End Results Program. Cancer stat facts—prostate cancer. 2019. Accessed May 20, 2020. https://seer.cancer.gov/statfacts /html/prost.html

10. National Institute of Mental Health. Men and depression. 2017.

11. SAVE (Suicide Awareness Voices of Education). Suicide facts. 2018. Accessed May 20, 2020. https://save.org/

12. Centers for Disease Control and Prevention. *National Diabetes Statistics Report 2020: Estimates of Diabetes and Its Burden in the United States.* 2020.

Chapter 3

1. Gardner B, Lally P, Wardle J. Making health habitual: the psychology of "habit formation" and general practice. *Br J Gen Pract.* 2012;664–666.

2. Mind Tools Content Team. Smart goals: how to make your goals achievable. Mind Tools. Accessed May 20, 2020. https://www.mindtools.com/pages/article/smart-goals.htm

Chapter 5

1. IQWiG. How does the prostate work? Informed Health. Updated 2019. https://www .informedhealth.org/how-does-the-prostate-work.2126.en.html

2. Lu S, Chen C. Natural history and epidemiology of benign prostatic hyperplasia. *Formosan Journal of Surgery.* 2014;207–210.

3. Ajayi A, Abraham K. Understanding the role of estrogen in the development of benign prostatic hyperplasia. *Afr J Urol.* 2018;93–97.

4. Carson C, Rittmaster R. The role of dihydrotestosterone in benign prostatic hyperplasia. *Urology.* 2003;2–7.

5. Lohsiriwat S, Hirunsai M, Chaiyaprasithi B. Effect of caffeine on bladder function in patients with overactive bladder symptoms. *Urol Ann.* 2011;3(1):14–18.

Chapter 6

1. American Cancer Society. Survival rates for prostate cancer. Updated 2019. https://www.cancer.org/cancer/prostate-cancer/detection-diagnosis-staging/survival-rates.html

2. American Cancer Society. Key statistics for prostate cancer. Updated 2019. https://www.cancer.org/cancer/prostate-cancer/about/key-statistics.html

3. Memorial Sloan Kettering Cancer Center. Hereditary cancer and genetics: inherited risk for prostate cancer. Updated 2019. https://www.mskcc.org/cancer-care/risk-assessment-screening/hereditary-genetics/genetic-counseling/inherited-risk-prostate

4. Chang ET, Boffetta P, Adami HO, Cole P, Mandel JS. A critical review of the epidemiology of agent orange/TCDD and prostate cancer. *Eur J Epidemiol.* 2014;667–723.

5. Huncharek M, Haddock KS, Reid R, Kupelnick B. Smoking as a risk factor for prostate cancer: a meta-analysis of 24 prospective cohort studies. *Am J Public Health.* 2010;693–701.

6. Demoury C, Karakiewicz P, Parent ME. Association between lifetime alcohol consumption and prostate cancer risk: a case-control study in Montreal, Canada. *Cancer Epidemiol.* 2016;11–17.

7. Muller RL, Faria EF, Carvalhal GF, Reis RB, Mauad EC, Carvalho AL, Freedland SJ. Association between family history of prostate cancer and positive biopsies in a Brazilian screening program. *World J Urol.* 2013;1273–1278.

8. Bratt O, Drevin L, Akre O, Garmo H, Stattin P. Family history and probability of prostate cancer, differentiated by risk category: a nationwide population-based study. *J Natl Cancer Inst.* 2016;108(10).

9. Bhindi B, Wallis CJD, Navan M, Farrell AM, Trost LW, Hamilton RJ, Kilkarni GS, Finelli A, Fleshner NE, Boorjian SA, Karnes RJ. The association between vasectomy and prostate cancer: a systematic review and meta-analysis. *JAMA Intern Med.* 2017;1273–1286.

10. Rider JR, Wilson KM, Sinnott JA, Kelly RS, Mucci LA, Giovannucci EL. Ejaculation frequency and risk of prostate cancer: updated results with an additional decade of follow-up. *Eur Urol.* 2016;974–982.

11. Prostate Cancer Foundation. The PSA test. Updated 2019. https://www.pcf.org/about-prostate-cancer/what-is-prostate-cancer/the-psa-test/

12. Samadi DB, Sebrow D, Hobbs AR, Bernstein AN, Brajtbord J, Lavery HJ, Jazayeri SB. Clinicopathological, functional, and immediate oncologic outcome assessment in men aged <50 years with prostate cancer after robotic prostatectomy. *Urol Oncol.* 2017;17–30. https://doi.org/10.1016/j.urolonc.2016.07.016

13. American Cancer Society. Survival rates for prostate cancer. Updated 2020. https://www.cancer.org/cancer/prostate-cancer/detection-diagnosis-staging/survival-rates.html

Chapter 7

1. Hirsch IH. *Structure of the Male Reproductive System.* Merck Manual Consumer Version. Revised 2017.

2. American Cancer Society. Cancer, sex and the male body. Updated 2019. https://www.cancer.org/treatment/treatments-and-side-effects/physical-side-effects/fertility-and-sexual-side-effects/sexuality-for-men-with-cancer/how-male-body-works-sexually.html

3. Feldman HA, Goldstein I, Hatzichristou DG, Krane RJ, McKinlay JB. Impotence and its medical and psychosocial correlates: results of the Massachusetts Male Aging Study. *J Urol.* 1994;54–61.

4. Kouidrat Y, Pizzol D, Cosco T, Thompson T, Carnaghi M, Bertoldo A, Solmi M, Stubbs B, Veronese N. High prevalence of erectile dysfunction in diabetes: a systematic review and meta-analysis of 145 studies. *Diabet Med.* 2017;1185–1192.

5. Hillier TA, Pedula KL. Complications in young adults with early-onset type 2 diabetes. *Diabetes Care.* 2003;2999–3005.

6. Sondhi M, Kakar A, Gogia A, Gupta M. Prevalence of erectile dysfunction in diabetic patients. *Curr Med Res Pract.* 2018;88–91.

7. Nunes KP, Labazi H, Webb RC. New insights into hypertension-associated erectile dysfunction. *Curr Opin Nephrol Hypertens.* 2012;163–170.

8. Hadi HA, Carr CS, Al Suwaidi J. Endothelial dysfunction: cardiovascular risk factors, therapy, and outcome. *Vasc Health Risk Manag.* 2005;183–198.

9. Chien YL, Pau-Chung C, Shyh-Chvi L, Pao-Ling T. The association of carotid intima-media thickness with serum level of perfluorinated chemicals and endothelium-platelet microparticles in adolescents and young adults. *Environ Int.* 2016;292–299.

10. Wu CH, Lu YY, Chai CY, Su YF, Tsai TH, Tsai FJ, Lin CL. Increased risk of osteoporosis in patients with erectile dysfunction: a nationwide population-based cohort study. *Medicine.* 2016;e4024.

11. Nur-Vaizura M, Ima-Nirwana S, Kok-Yong C. A concise review of testosterone and bone health. *Clin Interv Aging.* 2016;1317–1324.

12. Farag YMK, Guallar E, Zhao D, Kalyani RR, Blaha MJ, Feldman DI, Martin SS, Lutsey PL, Billups KL, Michos ED. Vitamin D deficiency is independently associated with greater prevalence of erectile dysfunction: the National Health and Nutrition Examination Survey (N-HANES) 2001–2004. *Atherosclerosis.* 2016;61–67.

13. Barassi A, Pezzilli R, Colpi GM, Massimiliano M, Gian Vico M. Vitamin D and erectile dysfunction. *J Sex Med.* 2014;2792–2800.

14. Mayo Clinic Laboratories. Test ID: TTFB testosterone, total, bioavailable, and free, serum. Accessed July 10, 2020. https://www.mayocliniclabs.com/test-catalog/Clinical+and+Interpretive/83686

15. Welliver RC, Wiser HJ, Brannigan RE, Feia K, Monga M, Kohler TS. Validity of midday total testosterone levels in older men with erectile dysfunction. *J Urol.* 2014. doi.org/10.1016/j.juro.2014.01.085

16. Brody S, Weiss P. Erectile dysfunction and premature ejaculation: interrelationships and psychosexual factors. *J Sex Med.* 2015;398–404.

17. Parnham A, Can Serefoglu E. Classification and definition of premature ejaculation. *Transl Androl Urol.* 2016;416–423.

18. American Cancer Society. Key statistics for penile cancer. Updated January 9, 2019. https://www.cancer.org/cancer/penile-cancer/about/key-statistics.html

19. Cancer.net. Testicular cancer: risk factors. 2019. Accessed July 10, 2020. https://www.cancer.net/cancer-types/testicular-cancer/risk-factors

20. Akar SZ, Bebis H. Evaluation of the effectiveness of testicular cancer and testicular self-examination training for patient care personnel: intervention study. *HEALTH EDUC RES.* 2014;29(6):966–976.

21. Morris BJ, Krieger JN. Penile inflammatory skin disorders and the preventive role of circumcision. *Int J Prev Med.* 2017;8(1):32.

22. Fakijan N, Hunter S, Cole GW, Miller J. An argument for circumcision: prevention of balanitis in the adult. *Arch Dermatol.* 1990;1046–1047.

Chapter 8

1. Sack H. Abraham Maslow and the hierarchy of needs. SciHi Blog. April 2015. http://scihi.org/tag/hierarchy-of-needs/

2. Charnetski CJ, Brennan F. Sexual frequency and salivary immunoglobulin A (IgA). *Psychol Rep.* 2004;839–44.

3. Frappier J, Toupin I, Levy J, Aubertin-Leheudre M, Karelis AD. Energy expenditure during sexual activity in young healthy couples. *PLoS One.* 2013;8(10):e79342.

4. Hambach A, Evers S, Summ O, Husstedt IW, Frese A. The impact of sexual activity on idiopathic headaches: an observational study. *Cephalalgia.* 2013;384–389.

5. Rider JR, Wilson KM, Sinnott JA, Kelly RS, Mucci LA, Giovannucci EL. Ejaculation frequency and risk of prostate cancer: updated results with an additional decade of follow-up. *Eur Urol.* 2016;974–982.

6. Hall SA, Shackelton R, Rosen RC, Araujo AB. Sexual activity, erectile dysfunction, and incident cardiovascular events. *Am J Cardiol.* 2010;192–197.

7. BBC News. Sex keeps you young. March 10, 1999. http://news.bbc.co.uk/2/hi/health/294119.stm

8. Centers for Disease Control and Prevention. Hepatitis B questions and answers for health professionals. Updated October 25, 2019. https://www.cdc.gov/hepatitis/hbv/hbvfaq.htm

9. Centers for Disease Control and Prevention. Genital herpes—CDC fact sheet. Updated August 28, 2017. https://www.cdc.gov/std/herpes/stdfact-herpes-detailed.htm

10. Resolve: The National Infertility Association. Fast facts on infertility. Updated 2017. https://resolve.org/infertility-101/what-is-infertility/fast-facts/

11. Chandra A, Copen CE. Infertility and impaired fecundity in the United States, 1982–2010: data from the National Survey of Family Growth. *National Health Statistics Reports.* Centers for Disease Control and Prevention. 2013;67:1–18.

12. Kovac JR, Khanna A, Lipshultz LI. The effects of cigarette smoking on male fertility. *Postgrad Med.* 2015;338–341.

13. Sheynkin Y, Jung M, Yoo P, Schulsinger D, Komaroff E. Increase in scrotal temperature in laptop computers users. *Hum Reprod.* 2005;452–455.

14. Agarwal A, Desai NR, Makker K, Varghese A, Mouradi R, Sabanegh E, Sharma R. Effects of radiofrequency electromagnetic waves (RD-EMW) from cellular phones on human ejaculated semen: an in vitro pilot study. *Fertil Steril.* 2009;1318–1325.

15. Giahi L, Mohammadmoradi S, Javidan A, Reza Sadeghi M. Nutritional modifications in male infertility: a systematic review covering 2 decades. *Nutr Rev.* 2016;118–130.

16. Levy R, Fezeu L, Faure C, Sermondade N, Sebastien C. Obesity and increased risk for oligozoospermia and azoospermia. *Arch Intern Med.* 2012;440–442.

17. Close CE, Roberts PL, Berger RE. Cigarettes, alcohol and marijuana are related to pyospermia in infertile men. *J Urol.* 1990;900–903.

18. Nassan FL, Arvizu M, Minguez-Alarcon L, Williams PL, et al. Marijuana smoking and markers of testicular function among men from a fertility centre. *Hum Reprod.* 2019;715–723.

19. Dorey G, Speakman MJ, Feneley RCL, Dunn CDR. Pelvic floor exercises for erectile dysfunction. *BJU Int.* 2005;96(4):595–597.

20. Pastore AL, Palleschi G, Fuschi A, Maggioni C, Rago R, Zucchi A, Costantini E, Carbone A. Pelvic floor muscle rehabilitation for patients with lifelong premature ejaculation: a novel therapeutic approach. *Ther Adv Urol.* 2014;83–88.

21. Emanuele MA, Emanuele NV. Alcohol's effects on male reproduction. *Alcohol Health Res World*. 1998;195–201.

22. Nolen-Hoeksema S. Gender differences in risk factors and consequences for alcohol use and problems. *Clin Psychol Rev*. 2004;981–1010.

23. Kovac JR, Labbate C, Ramasamy R, Tang D, Lipshultz LI. Effects of cigarette smoking on erectile dysfunction. *Andrologia*. 2015;1087–1092.

24. Pereira Antoniassi M, Intasqui P, Camargo M, Suslik Zylbersztein D, Melechco Carvalho V, Cardoza KHM, Pimenta Bertolla R. Analysis of the functional aspects and seminal plasma proteomic profile of sperm from smokers. *BJU Int*. 2016;118(5):814–822.

Chapter 9

1. The Food Industry Association. Supermarket facts. Updated 2018. https://www.fmi.org /our-research/supermarket-facts

2. Reynolds A, Mann J, Cummings J, Winter N, Mete E, Te Morengo L. Carbohydrate quality and human health: a series of systematic reviews and meta-analyses. *Lancet*. 2019;434–445.

3. Valdes AM, Walter J, Segal E, Spector TD. Role of the gut microbiota in nutrition and health. *BMJ*. 2018;361:k2179.

4. David L, Maurice C, Carmody R, et al. Diet rapidly and reproducibly alters the human gut microbiome. *Nature*. 2014;505:559–563.

5. U.S. Department of Health and Human Services. Appendix 7: Nutrition goals for age-sex groups based on dietary reference intakes and dietary guidelines recommendations. Updated 2011. https://health.gov/our-work/food-nutrition/2015-2020-dietary-guidelines /guidelines/appendix-7/

6. Xie J, de Souza AV, von der Haar T, Coldwell MJ, Wang X, Proud CG. Regulation of the elongation phase of protein synthesis enhances translation accuracy and modulates lifespan. *Curr Biol*. February 2019.

7. Paddon-Jones D, Campbell WW, Jacques PF, Kritchevsky SB, Moore LL, Rodriguez NR, van Loon LJC. Protein and healthy aging. *Am J Clin Nutr*. 2015;1339S–1345S.

8. U.S. Food and Drug Administration. Final determination regarding partially hydrogenated oils (removing trans fat). Updated 2018. https://www.fda.gov/food/food-additives-petitions /final-determination-regarding-partially-hydrogenated-oils-removing-trans-fat

9. Guasch-Ferre M, Liu X, Malik VS, Sun O, Willett WC, Manson JE, Rexrode KM, Li Y, Hu FB, Bhupathiraiu SN. Nut consumption and risk of cardiovascular disease. *J Am Coll Cardiol*. 2017;70(20).

10. World Health Organization. Q&A on the carcinogenicity of the consumption of red meat and processed meat. Updated 2015. https://www.who.int/news-room/q-a-detail/q-a-on -the-carcinogenicity-of-the-consumption-of-red-meat-and-processed-meat

11. Council for Responsible Nutrition. Dietary supplement use reaches all time high— available-for-purchase consumer survey reaffirms the vital role supplementation plays in the lives of most Americans. Updated 2019. https://www.crnusa.org/newsroom /dietary-supplement-use-reaches-all-time-high

12. NPR. Vitamin D and fish oil supplements mostly disappoint in long-awaited research results. Updated 2018. https://www.npr.org/sections/health-shots/2018/11/10/666545527 /vitamin-d-and-fish-oil-supplements-disappoint-in-long-awaited-study-results

13. Risk and Prevention Study Collaborative Group, Roncaglioni MC, Tombesi M, et al. n-3 fatty acids in patients with multiple cardiovascular risk factors. *N Engl J Med.* 2013;368:1800–1808.

14. National Cancer Institute. Selenium and vitamin E cancer prevention trial (SELECT): questions and answers. Updated 2015. https://www.cancer.gov/types/prostate/research/select-trial-results-qa

Chapter 10

1. Young SN. How to increase serotonin in the human brain without drugs. *J Psychiatry Neurosci.* 2007;394–399.

2. Chowdhury R, Guitart-Masip M, Bunzeck N, Dolan RJ, Duzel E. Dopamine modulates episodic memory persistence in old age. *J Neurosci.* 2012;14193–14204.

3. Oppezzo M, Schwartz DL. Give your ideas some legs: the positive effect of walking on creative thinking. *Journal of Experimental Psychology: Learning, Memory, and Cognition.* 2014;1142–1152.

4. Colzato LS, Szapora A, Pannekoek JN, Hommel B. The impact of physical exercise on convergent and divergent thinking. *Front Hum Neurosci.* 2013. doi.org/10.3389/fnhum.2013.00824

5. Thompson Coon J, Boddy K, Stein K, Whear R, Barton J, Depledge MH. Does participating in physical activity in outdoor natural environments have a greater effect on physical and mental wellbeing than physical activity indoors? a systematic review. *Environ Sci Technol.* 2011;1761–1772.

6. Blackwell DL, Clarke TC. State variation in meeting the 2008 federal guidelines for both aerobic and muscle-strengthening activities through leisure-time physical activity among adults aged 18–64: United States, 2010–2015. *Natl Health Stat Report.* 2018;(112):1–22.

7. U.S. Department of Health and Human Services. *Physical Activity Guidelines.* Updated 2019. https://www.hhs.gov/fitness/be-active/physical-activity-guidelines-for-americans/index.html

8. Piercy KL, Trojano RP, Ballard RM, et al. The physical activity guidelines for Americans. *JAMA Network.* 2018;2020–2028.

9. Bushman B. Promoting exercise as medicine for prediabetes and prehypertension. *Curr Sports Med Rep.* 2014;13:233–239.

10. Sousa N, Mendes R, Abrantes C, Sampaio J, Oliveira J. A randomized study on lipids response to different exercise programs in overweight older men. *Int J Sports Med.* 2014;35:1106–1111.

11. Janssen I, Katzmarzyk PT, Ross R, Leon AS, Skinner JS, Rao DC, et al. Fitness alters the associations of BMI and waist circumference with total and abdominal fat. *Obesity.* 2004;12:523–537.

12. Van Dijk JW, Venema M, van Mechelen W, Stehouwer CD, Hartgen F, van Loon LL. Effect of moderate-intensity exercise versus activities of daily living on 24-hour blood glucose homeostasis in male patients with type 2 diabetes. *Diabetes Care.* 2013;36:3448–3453.

13. U.S. Department of Health and Human Services. *2018 Physical Activity Guidelines for Americans.* Updated 2019. https://www.hhs.gov/fitness/be-active/physical-activity-guidelines-for-americans/index.html

14. Tucker, LA, Strong JE, Lecheminant JD, Bailey BW. Effect of two jumping programs on hip bone mineral density in premenopausal women: a randomized controlled trial. *Am J Health Promot.* 2015;158–164.

15. Menicucci D, Piarulli A, Mastorci F, Sebastiani L, et al. Interactions between immune, stress-related hormonal and cardiovascular systems following strenuous physical exercise. *Arch Ital Biol.* 2013;126–136.

16. U.S. Department of Health and Human Services. *2018 Physical Activity Guidelines Scientific Report.* Updated 2018. https://health.gov/our-work/physical-activity/current-guidelines/scientific-report

17. Akbari Kamrani AA, Shams A, Shamsipour Dehkordi P, Mohajeri R. The effect of low and moderate-intensity aerobic exercises on sleep quality in male older adults. *Pak J Med Sci.* 2014;417–421.

Chapter 11

1. National Sleep Foundation. National Sleep Foundation recommends new sleep times. Updated 2015. https://www.sleepfoundation.org/press-release/national-sleep-foundation-recommends-new-sleep-times

2. Shlisky JD, Hartman TJ, Kris-Etherton PM, Rogers CJ, Sharkey NA, Nickols-Richardson SM. Partial sleep deprivation and energy balance in adults: an emerging issue for consideration by dietetic practitioners. *J Acad Nutr Diet.* 2012;1785–1797.

3. American Psychological Association. 2015 Stress in America. Updated 2015. https://www.apa.org/news/press/releases/stress/

4. Kaiser Family Foundation. The implications of COVID-19 on mental health and substance abuse. Accessed May 22, 2020. https://www.kff.org/coronavirus-covid-19/issue-brief/the-implications-of-covid-19-for-mental-health-and-substance-use/

INDEX

Made in United States
Orlando, FL
19 August 2022

21294823R00141